Video-Reflexive Ethnography in Health Research and Healthcare Improvement

Video-Reflexive Ethnography in Health Research and Healthcare Improvement

Theory and Application

Rick Iedema
King's College London, London, UK

Katherine Carroll
Australian National University, Canberra, Australia

Aileen Collier
University of Auckland, Auckland, New Zealand

Su-yin Hor
University of Technology, Sydney, Australia

Jessica Mesman
Maastricht University, Maastricht, The Netherlands

Mary Wyer
The Westmead Institute for Medical Research, Westmead, Australia

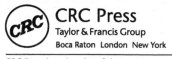

CRC Press
Taylor & Francis Group
Boca Raton London New York

CRC Press is an imprint of the
Taylor & Francis Group, an **informa** business

CRC Press
Taylor & Francis Group
6000 Broken Sound Parkway NW, Suite 300
Boca Raton, FL 33487-2742

© 2019 by Taylor & Francis Group, LLC
CRC Press is an imprint of Taylor & Francis Group, an Informa business

No claim to original U.S. Government works

Printed on acid-free paper

International Standard Book Number-13: 978-0-8153-7035-2 (Hardback)
International Standard Book Number-13: 978-0-8153-7033-8 (Paperback)

Library of Congress Cataloging-in-Publication Data

Names: Iedema, Rick, author. | Carroll, Katherine (Health care researcher), author. | Collier, Aileen, author. | Hor, Su-yin, author. | Mesman, Jessica, 1962- author. | Wyer, Mary (Mary S.), author.
Title: Video reflexive ethnography in health research and healthcare improvement: a practical guide / by Rick Iedema, Katherine Carroll, Aileen Collier, Su-yin Hor, Jessica Mesman and Mary Wyer.
Description: First edition. | Boca Raton, FL: CRC Press ; Taylor & Francis Group, [2019] | Includes bibliographical references and index.
Identifiers: LCCN 2018033075| ISBN 9780815370338 (pbk.: alk. paper) | ISBN 9780815370352 (hardback: alk. paper) | ISBN 9781351248013 (ebook).
Subjects: LCSH: Medical care—Research—Methodology. | Video recording in ethnology.
Classification: LCC RA440.85 .I34 2019 | DDC 362.1072—dc23
LC record available at https://lccn.loc.gov/2018033075

Visit the Taylor & Francis Web site at
http://www.taylorandfrancis.com

and the CRC Press Web site at
http://www.crcpress.com

Contents

Authors

Rick Iedema is a Professor and the Director of the Centre for Team-based Practice and Learning in Health Care, King's College London, London, United Kingdom.

Katherine Carroll is a Research Fellow in the School of Sociology, Australian National University, Canberra, Australia.

Aileen Collier is Senior Lecturer, Te Arai Palliative Care and End of Life Research Group, School of Nursing, Faculty of Medicine and Health Sciences, University of Auckland, New Zealand.

Su-yin Hor is a Lecturer in Health Services Management, Faculty of Health, University of Technology Sydney, Sydney, Australia.

Jessica Mesman is an Associate Professor, Department of Society Studies, Maastricht University, Maastricht, the Netherlands.

Mary Wyer is a Postdoctoral Researcher at the Centre for Infectious Diseases and Microbiology, The Westmead Institute for Medical Research, Westmead, New South Wales, Australia.

Introduction

0.0 VIDEO-REFLEXIVE ETHNOGRAPHY AS PRACTICE

We start this book with a vignette to provide an example of video-reflexive ethnography (VRE) as practice (Iedema et al., 2015):

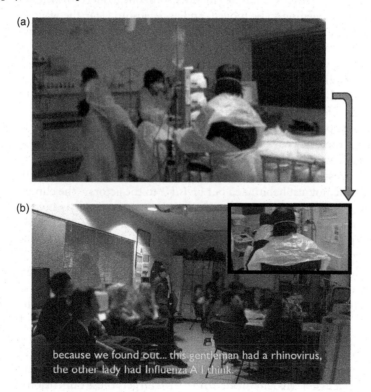

Figure 0.1 (a) Clinicians in sterile gowns and gloves pushing an infectious patient through the intensive care unit. (b) Clinicians observing footage of how they push an infectious patient through the intensive care unit. The arrow points to the original footage being shown to the clinicians (in the box in the top right corner) while they're discussing this footage.

The image in Figure 0.1a is taken from a video clip that was filmed during a project on infection control practices. The clinicians in the clip are wheeling a bed through an intensive care unit (ICU), and they are wearing gowns and gloves so as to protect themselves from the patient's pathogens. The patient in the bed has rhinovirus and needs to be moved to an isolation room to prevent other patients becoming infected. As the bed is wheeled through the ICU, the clinicians encounter different obstacles, among them an X-ray machine, which needs to be pushed out of the way. Given that every one of them is potentially contaminated with the patient's pathogens, touching these obstacles encourages cross-contamination.

Figure 0.1b shows an inset box that displays the original footage, and the rest of the image shows the clinicians viewing that footage and engaging in practice reflexivity. When they were given the opportunity to reflect on this event using video footage in this way, the clinicians realized that their touching ICU technologies and instruments may have compromised the barrier precautions that they set out to achieve. As they reviewed the footage of this event, they talk about how to prevent similar problems from re-occurring. Could they prepare their trajectory better? Could they identify someone to alert other ICU clinicians to the patient needing to be moved, and ask them to clear the way? Could they anticipate these kinds of problems better by thinking ahead, and by planning their activities in smarter ways?

The above vignette highlights the essentials of VRE. Using VRE, we approach care as a locally unfolding dynamic process. This process is captured on video and prepared for feedback in the form of short clips. Participants in the process and their colleagues are invited to review the resulting footage. Their involvement in this process serves the purpose of enabling them to identify the aspects of practice that they have started to treat as given – that is, seeing their activities as normal, natural and necessary.

The expression 'taken-as-given' is often used in VRE to refer to activities that have become not just habituated but *invisible* to the actors – the clinicians or the patients – themselves. While not all our habits are necessarily invisible to ourselves, some we have learned to find no longer remarkable. These are the habits we now treat as normal, natural and necessary. These are the habits that we tend to justify in the face of challenges because they provide anchorage for who we are and how we are with others. In short, these are habits that we have decided or learned *to forget*.

VRE invites professionals and patients to approach care as that which results from our actions and intentions, as well as from habits that we no longer see reason to question. Our activity harbours many such habits, and such habits may underpin activities that are suboptimal. VRE grants us opportunities to reassess and reshape precisely those dimensions of our own behaviour that otherwise remain inaccessible (Iedema et al., 2013). VRE targets these dimensions of human behaviour because they define, shape and constrain how everyday care unfolds. Where other endeavours regard behaviour as a manifestation of professional culture or personal psychology, VRE approaches it as a facet of practice – that is, of how people are and work together. VRE targets behaviour on the view that people rarely get the opportunity to scrutinize themselves and each other in action, and that this denies them the opportunity to reshape their behaviour, to become more intelligent about their behaviour and to orient their behaviour better to the exigencies of everyday patient care.

The remainder of this chapter introduces this book and its contents. This chapter will also expand on the role and rationale of VRE in relation to the existing healthcare research literature, and the relevant theoretical and methodological literatures. Finally, the chapter will explain how to navigate the applied and theoretical contents of the book, before finishing with an overview of each of the book's chapters.

0.1 WHY THIS BOOK?

The field of healthcare improvement includes endeavours as varied as patient safety research, quality of care research, clinical practice improvement, health service research, health policy reform and implementation science. This book keys in to this array of endeavours in the following ways: first, without tying itself to any one of these types of research and improvement, VRE may unfold in ways that have relevance for one or more of the endeavours just listed. This is because VRE is agnostic about how to label an aspect of practice on which front-line professionals and their researchers or facilitators may decide to concentrate. Using VRE to address different staff members' understandings about and approaches to using clean and sterile gloves, for example, may have relevance for patients' safety, for the implementation of infection control (and hand hygiene) guidelines, for practice improvement and so on.

Second, most endeavours that are currently in use to achieve improvements in health care start with the assumption that specialized knowledge must be the first step towards change. These endeavours operate on the principle that specialists and experts are needed to produce formalized knowledge about what is going on. An example of such specialized knowledge is 'statistical process control' (Hart and Hart, 2002), which is a statistical analysis of everyday processes relying on numerical data about patients' movements, bed occupation and so forth. Such knowledge is reliant on elaborate kinds of reporting and analysis, and its conclusions need 'translating' back into everyday practice. This knowledge translation model is ubiquitous across most if not all areas of healthcare improvement, quality, safety and so forth. To be sure, the knowledge translation model may be suited to the improvement of those facets of care that are relatively technical and automated. Here, we can think of the more or less standardized dimensions of pharmacy, radiotherapy and nuclear medicine (Vincent and Amalberti, 2016). We acknowledge that even these three areas can be complex – think, for example, of pharmaceutical practices in palliative care which are far from simple and standardized. Yet such areas may nevertheless be amenable to being structured and organized according to generalized and more or less stable knowledge.

While few if any aspects of medicine are fully iterative and mechanical, and few are completely chaotic, some are definitely more complex than others. For example, both paediatric and geriatric patients are now displaying quite complex disease patterns due to our ability to raise life chances for a greater number of patients. A paediatrician who attended one of our classes recently said, 'On my wards I see increasing numbers of young patients with respiratory problems that are so complex that I feel unsure about not just how to treat them. I am also unsure about how to teach students on placements about what is going on in my ward'. The complexity that is inherent in these patients' care means that professionals increasingly face care situations where novel ways of moving forward need to be devised and negotiated. This means that generalized knowledge now increasingly needs to be contextualized with knowledge of local circumstances, contextual constraints and emergent opportunities. The people who have access to these latter kinds of knowledge are not necessarily clinical specialists or experts, but people who know about patients' situations and who understand what may be necessary or preferable (Fitzsimons and Cornwell, 2018). Here, we can think about how we negotiate patients' end of life, about where and how they die and about whose knowledge and priorities are made to count (Collier, 2013).

Third, VRE is deliberately oriented towards giving front-line professionals and patients a say in what needs to be the focus of researchers' and practice improvers' attention. This 'democratic' underpinning of VRE will reappear as a theme throughout this book. For now, we will only note that this democratic orientation is not 'just' politically or ethically motivated, even though that in itself would be more than justified. Indeed, you listen to front-line clinicians and patients talking about day-to-day care, or observe what goes on moment to moment in primary care practices, hospital wards, medical specialties and anywhere else where care occurs, and you realize that front-line professionals' and patients' wealth of experience and insight deserves to be made more central to how we think about everything from safety and quality to improvement, implementation and policy reform.

Importantly, VRE's democratic orientation is also *theoretically* and *methodologically* motivated. We want to involve professionals and patients at the frontline of care because they are the people who are experiencing the complexity of *in situ* care more than anyone else. In fact, we can put it like this: theoretically as well as practically speaking, *in situ* care is the zone of maximum complexity. Experts may talk about 'complex adaptive systems' that they describe as happening beyond your reach, but these are hypotheses or imputations. We, by contrast, hold the view that complexity happens in the 'here and now' of care, even if this complexity comes about as a result of innumerable influences whose origin may lie elsewhere. If we fail to meet the 4-hour rule in the emergency department, it may have to do with how ambulances are routed, with last year's staffing decisions, with primary care referral habits or with 30-year-old corridor widths and ward designs preventing appropriate oversight over patient cohorts. The manifestation of these things occurs in and around the care of patients in the here and now.

Enabling those embroiled in these situations to step back and identify the sources of stress, and, if necessary, to look beyond ward and service boundaries, is critical to addressing situational complexity. But 'the world is seen in a grain of sand' (Blake, 1863), and too often do we ignore the sand around our feet in preference to impressive sounding promises of better shores.

0.2 OUR LEADING THESIS

This then is the leading thesis of this book: *in situ* care is the zone of maximum complexity. Front-line clinicians and patients and their families inhabit this zone of maximum complexity day in and day out. By the same token, experts, researchers, business consultants and managers tend not to be party to that zone of maximum complexity, because they don't work there and spend little to no time there. They may wield symbols and representations about care (in the form of reports, data, statistics and narratives), but symbols and representations do not equal lived reality. Put differently, 'the map is not the territory' (to use a phrase coined by Alfred Korzybski (Kodish, 2011)). What the map lacks is a rich experiential dimension that only comes to life when we participate in the day-to-day unfolding of care.

To be sure, we do not want to dismiss the significance of analyses based on reported data, or of guidelines derived from such analyses setting out courses of action, or of expertise anchored in experience expressed through narratives or consensus guidelines. Yet we are conscious that contemporary care is frequently so complex that professionals and patients are more often now than ever obliged to update the ways they do care and devise novel ways of moving forward. A patient may wish to die only after having glimpsed the ocean. Parents of a severely disabled baby may wish for the baby to be kept alive against the advice of doctors. Collectively, professionals, managers, service users, policy makers and the public are now obliged to contemplate and venture into new domains where they may have to consider doing the not-yet-done, saying the not-yet-said or thinking the not-yet-thought.

This last point positions front-line professionals and patients as critical players in everything we do in health care: they inhabit this zone of maximum complexity. Admittedly this maxim – 'frontline professionals and patients are critical players in healthcare improvement' – is becoming increasingly prominent now in healthcare reform, health services improvement and implementation research. Clinicians are indeed more and more involved in practice improvement in one way or another; patients are surveyed and interviewed to within an inch of their lives, and outcome measures are now structured to reflect everyday experiential as well as clinical-technical priorities (e.g. 'patient reported outcome and experience measures').

But the everyday experiences of professionals and patients are not yet commonly or comprehensively allowed to inform or structure healthcare improvements, implementation programmes or healthcare policy reforms. People's narratives are becoming more prominent in online websites, interview quotes are now sprinkled throughout reports and videoed comments are more prominent in formal presentations. But only rarely do front-line professionals and patients get the chance to articulate and shape their views, feelings, ideas and insights together, and negotiate what is good and what may need to be changed, and how and why, *on their terms*.

0.3 VRE AS NOVEL PARADIGM

We outlined the reasons for why VRE turns existing paradigms on their head. VRE's point of departure is the view that front-line professionals and patients and their families know everyday care by living it every day. They inhabit the zone of maximum complexity. They are a critical source of insight into the local ecology of care provision that unfolds there. The term 'ecology' refers to the complex historical, local and contextual facets of how care is provided by specific services. Each service is different due to the different ways in which technologies, guidelines, pathways and policies are put to use. Local people know their own services like no other, and their knowledge is critical to rethinking how care is to be provided. Their knowledge may not always be explicit and articulate, but it will certainly be fully embodied and deeply sensed (Iedema et al., 2018). VRE capitalizes on their experiences, feelings and insights.

VRE is further different from other improvement approaches because it acknowledges that 'life is outrunning the pedagogies in which we have been trained' (Fisher, 2003: 37). We have grown up with closely held assumptions about knowledge, authority and value that may no longer be in sync with the modern world. The modern world moves too fast for us to maintain old ways of knowing and learning. We need new approaches to running and shaping our lives, routines, habits and practices, because leaving these things to chance is now too risky (Iedema et al., 2018). For that reason, VRE presents a new research paradigm that functions as pedagogy, as a new way of learning about the world, starting from everyday *in situ* care and from those who populate and embody that care.

Giving primacy to 'what is', and to those populating it, VRE does not seek out specific kinds of data to suit specific kinds of analysis, other than footage and actors' interpretations of that footage. In that sense, VRE is not so much a qualitative methodology, as a 'post-qualitative' form of inquiry (Lather and St. Pierre, 2013). For St. Pierre, post-qualitative *inquiry* or *research* moves away from linear programmes and methodological rigidity, towards more creative approaches that allow for more possibilities in understanding and reshaping practice (St. Pierre, 2014).

As post-qualitative methodology (Wyer et al., 2017), VRE is open to different levels of participant–researcher engagement (Carroll, 2009). VRE produces video footage *and* reflexive discussion about 'what goes on', in collaboration with those who inhabit practices and services, the professionals and patients and their families. VRE's success depends on these stakeholders' enthusiasm and participation, but it welcomes a wide array of researcher–participant configurations (Carroll and Mesman, 2018).

Likewise, VRE may involve upfront agenda setting ('This project is about infection control', or 'We'd like to work with you on your clinical handovers'), or it may be fully clinician- and patient-driven (Iedema and Merrick, 2008). VRE may position the researcher(s) as the person(s) to select the resulting footage, or this selection may occur on the advice of, or be entirely under the control of, clinician participants. We, by no means, dismiss the significance and challenges of working through these kinds of decisions and negotiations, and they will be addressed in detail throughout what follows. For now, we will only state as ideal that VRE hands the reins as much as is practically possible to those professionals and patients who regard viewing footage of their practices as an opportunity to enhance their agency in relation to how care is done from moment to moment.

Most likely, those who participate in VRE projects are people interested in exploring their own roles and responsibilities for how care happens in the here and now. They are people who are adventurous enough to do so. They essentially venture into a zone where the complexity of the 'here and now' is framed as a dimension of how they are with one another, how they work with one another, how they speak to one another, how they organize care together and how they feel about one another. This zone also confronts them with the aspects of their behaviour that may be below their level of awareness: (how) do they perform the expectations that are inherent in their organization's culture, systems, rules, identities, relationships and practices (Iedema et al., 2018)? They are people who are open to acknowledging that changing anything in health care is contingent on whether and how they can connect the change to their existing ways of working, and whether they regard the change as logical, reasonable, warranted, feasible and understood in similar ways by those with whom they work.

This brings us to the end of our initial introductory statement. Each of the points made here will be revisited in the chapters that follow. We will provide examples and offer advice based on the many studies we have thus far conducted and are currently conducting. What remains most central in all of this, however, is our basic philosophy, which can now be summarized and expressed in terms of the following four themes.

First, *in situ* care is the zone of maximal complexity. Clinicians and patients are most closely involved in care: they *embody* this complexity, and they are therefore the people who are critical to learning about and intervening in that complexity. Second, as outsiders and 'alongsiders' (Carroll, 2009), we the researchers collaborate with front-line professionals, patients and their families, in their quest to illuminate the ecology and complexity of care. Third, engaging professionals, patients and their families with footage of everyday care practices gives them the opportunity to reflect on and clarify what they do, how they do it and why they do it. Fourth, all this is contingent on the (psychological) safety of VRE participants. This safety results not just from being respected for adopting a reflexive stance but also from stakeholders in the service and the wider system respecting and acting on the wisdom embodied and articulated through this process.

In the remaining chapters, we frame these themes in the form of four principles: *exnovation, collaboration, reflexivity,* and *care.* The term 'exnovation' was promoted first in our 2013 book on VRE (Iedema et al., 2013). There, we explained the importance of front-line professionals themselves focusing on their practices, and thereby deriving and designing change. This bottom-up process we referred to as exnovation, to contrast it with innovation, or expert-directed change imposed from the outside or from the top down. The term 'exnovation' combines excavation with innovation: looking more closely at what is to identify opportunities for change, rather than looking farther afield for solutions.

Collaboration undergirds VRE in that professionals and patients are invited as participants from the moment an initiative or project is to be conceived. They are experts in the everyday unfolding of care, and their habits, assumptions and expectations are the anchors of that care.

For its part, reflexivity is central to VRE also. Reflexivity is to be distinguished from reflection. We regard reflection as a personal activity that focuses the individual on their past thoughts and actions. Reflexivity, by contrast, is a shared, social deliberation about existing circumstances and practices such that these are apprehended from new perspectives and in new ways. This creates the possibility not just for new insights but also for new identities and new social and organizational realities (Iedema, 2011).

Finally, care is the pre-condition of VRE per se. Without care, the collaborative, creative and practical dimensions of VRE cannot be realized. Participants need to feel safe, respected and valued to devote themselves to scrutinizing footage of their own ways of working, and to speaking openly, honestly and creatively about their own assumptions, habits, values and views. These four principles have important implications – methodological, political and ethical – and we will touch on these throughout the book.

0.4 CONTENTS OF THE BOOK

Chapter 1 is designed for academic audiences who are interested in the theoretical links and underpinnings of VRE. Chapter 2 equips you with the necessary tools, processual knowledge and tips to fund, plan and obtain ethics approval for VRE in a healthcare setting. Chapter 3 focuses on participant recruitment for VRE projects, videoing processes and practices and the role of visual analysis in VRE. Chapter 4 prepares you for the techniques and strategies that are at the heart of videoing *in situ* practices. Chapters 5 and 6 focus on the dynamics and facilitation of video-reflexive sessions. Chapter 7 describes the challenge of evaluating VRE projects and achievements. Chapter 8 addresses the issues that arise when you want to publish or present about your VRE project. Chapter 9 concludes the book by returning to the more theoretical and philosophical underpinnings of VRE.

REFERENCES

Blake W. (1863) Auguries of Innocence. Poerty Foundation. URL: https://www. poetryfoundation.org/poems/43650/auguries-of-innocence

Carroll K. (2009) Insider, outsider, alongsider: Examining reflexivity in hospital based video research. *International Journal for Multiple Research Approaches* 3: 246–263.

Carroll K and Mesman J. (2018) Multiple researcher roles in video-reflexive ethnography. *Qualitative Health Research* 28: 1145–1156.

Collier A. (2013) Deleuzians of patient safety: A video reflexive ethnography of end of life care. PhD Thesis. Sydney: Centre for Health Communication, University of Technology Sydney.

Fisher M. (2003) *Emergent Forms of Life and the Anthropological Voice.* Durham, NC: Duke University Press.

Fitzsimons B and Cornwell J. (2018) What can we learn from patients' perspectives on the quality and safety of hospital care? *BMJ Quality & Safety* 27: 673–682.

Hart MK and Hart RF. (2002) *Statistical Process Control for Health Care.* Pacific Grove, CA: Duxbury.

Iedema R. (2011) Creating safety by strengthening clinicians' capacity for reflexivity. *BMJ Quality and Safety* 20: S83–S86.

Iedema R, Hor S, Wyer M, et al. (2015) An innovative approach to strengthening health professionals' infection control and limiting hospital acquired infection: video-reflexive ethnography. *BMJ Innovation.* doi:10.1136/bmjinnov-2014-000032.

Iedema R, Jorm C, Hor S, et al. (2018) To follow a rule? On frontline clinicians' understandings and embodiments of hospital-acquired infection prevention and control rules. *Health.* doi:10.1177/1363459318785677.

Iedema R and Merrick E. (2008) 'Handover – Enabling Learning in Communication for Safety (HELiCS)' – A DVD/Booklet-based Kit for Handover Improvement. Sydney: Australian Commission on Safety and Quality in Health Care & University of Technology Sydney.

Iedema R, Mesman J, and Carroll K. (2013) *Visualising Health Care Improvement: Innovation from Within,* Oxford: Radcliffe.

Kodish BI. (2011) *Korzybski: A Biography.* Pasadena: Extensional Publishing.

Lather P and St. Pierre EA. (2013) Post-qualitative research. *International Journal of Qualitative Studies in Education* 26: 629–633.

St. Pierre E. (2014) A brief and personal history of post qualitative research: Toward 'post inquiry'. *Journal of Curriculum Theorizing* 30: 2–19.

Vincent C and Amalberti R. (2016) *Safer Healthcare: Strategies for the Real World.* Heidelberg: Springer.

Wyer M, Iedema R, Hor S, et al. (2017) Patient involvement can affect clinicians' perspectives and practices of infection prevention and control: A 'post-qualitative' study using video-reflexive ethnography. *International Journal of Qualitative Research Methods* 16: 1–10.

1

The theoretical background of video-reflexive ethnography

1.1 INTRODUCTION

This chapter presents the theoretical bases for the more practical-focused chapters that follow. It details the four basic principles that are at the heart of video-reflexive ethnography (VRE): exnovation, collaboration, reflexivity and care. It also explains how video accesses the everyday dimensions of care, and why doing so is important for unveiling and tackling the complexity of care. This further includes a discussion about the locus of complexity, arguing that complexity and complex systems are not some specialized realms of reality to which only experts have adequate access. On the contrary, we argue that complexity and complex systems are available to us and tangible for us depending on how we view and construe the world, and on what we want to achieve in the world.

As will become apparent throughout this book, VRE has been applied to a wide range and variety of topics and healthcare settings. Its applications range from improving clinical practices (such as handovers and infection control) in hospital wards to exploring what respect means in clinical consultations between patients and doctors, and what safety means for dying patients in palliative care contexts. The flexibility of VRE is undergirded by a theoretical framework that describes how and why VRE uses video to intervene in everyday healthcare practices, to analyze these practices *reflexively* and in *collaboration* with stakeholders – who may be clinicians, patients, health services managers, or ancillary staff. Of course, you may skip the present theoretical chapter if you are interested purely in VRE's practical application. However, understanding VRE's theoretical basis may strengthen your methodological decision-making in whatever setting you are interested in, for whatever topic, and with whomever your collaborators and participants are.

This flexibility forms an important part of VRE. Rather than prescribing a set of methods and procedures, we recommend instead a methodology that is essentially a way of 'doing with theory' (Jackson and Mazzei, 2012). In other words, VRE is a 'methodology-to-come' as it relies on you creatively applying the principles set out in this chapter to the situation at hand.

> There is no methodological instrumentality to be unproblematically learned. In this methodology-to-come, we begin to do it differently wherever we are in our projects.
>
> *(Lather, 2013: 635)*

Let's now turn to the four guiding principles underlying VRE: exnovation, collaboration, reflexivity and care. We will detail how the use of video realizes these principles. To this end, we draw on theoretical arguments from fields including practice theory, science and technology studies, participatory action research, feminist research and education.

As indicated in the introduction to this book, these four guiding principles for VRE and their rationales are as follows:

1. *Exnovation*: VRE foregrounds the local ecology of care, that is, the accomplishment and complexity of everyday and taken-as-given care practices unfolding in the here and now.
2. *Collaboration*: VRE is a participatory approach to data co-creation, analysis and redesign with stakeholders, since they are steeped in the local ecology of care.
3. *Reflexivity*: VRE enables and encourages participants (professionals, patients) to re-view and re-imagine their practices, since they carry within them a deep (if not always articulate) sense of what is deemed appropriate and what is now possible; VRE also motivates reflexivity on the part of the researcher(s) since it puts their practice(s) at risk too.
4. *Care*: VRE cares for participants' (psychological) safety as they delve into care complexity, and VRE credits participants' contributions with relevance and significance for intervening in that complexity.

Video-reflexive ethnographers work to make visible and intervene in the complexity of mundane everyday activity. They do so through a process that is referred to as *exnovation* (principle 1). This commitment to engaging with complexity requires us to attend to care practices as they unfold *in situ*. Since front-line clinicians and patients are closest to care as it unfolds *in situ*, researchers work closely with local actors (principle 2) to create video footage of them enacting these everyday practices. This also means that the activity normally called data collection is more like a 'co-creation' of meaning, resources and attention. Likewise, analysis is principally a form of reflexivity (principle 3) – that is, a process of making sense of practices as *embedded within* their contexts (Bleakley, 1999). This reflexivity emerges through and from the questioning discussions among participants in response to viewing footage. It applies to professionals, researchers *and* patients. In fact, reflexivity is likely to occur at multiple points during a VRE project, and it informs the ongoing sense-making decisions about what to video, what to show back, and how to organize and facilitate reflexive discussions. This sense-making drives how we negotiate relationships and monitors appropriate levels of care for participants (principle 4).

This fourth principle attends to the understanding that there is a potential for feelings of shame and vulnerability to arise from improvement activities. Particularly, since improvement questions tend to be put among co-workers, others' perception that someone's performance is below par may give that person the feeling that 'however good your performance has been, it is not as good as it could be' (Davidoff, 2002: 2). In VRE, the risk of adverse effect is accentuated by the potential for video to be used for performance monitoring and risk mitigation. This may exacerbate vulnerable participants' lack of power and control over their own and organizational circumstances (such as patients or less powerful healthcare workers). For this reason, VRE sets great store by the principle to *care* for our participants and ourselves, and ensures their and our psychological safety (Edmondson, 1999, 2002). Care is critical to ensuring that everyone feels safe taking risks by having his/her video-recorded behaviours viewed, edited and scrutinized by others, and speaking up about his/her own and others' practices, without being embarrassed, rejected or punished.

We address the first three principles – exnovation, collaboration, and reflexivity, in the present chapter. We elaborate the fourth principle, care, in the chapter that follows, Chapter 2.

In the following sections, we discuss how video facilitates the contextual 'closeness' described previously and how video-reflexivity requires the kinds of collaboration that are less about researchers and participants cooperating from discrete positions of expertise, and more about the blurring of boundaries such that participants become co-researchers, and researchers become co-participants (Goodyear-Smith et al., 2015). This use of video may even lead to situations where researchers are no longer needed to inspire professionals to observe themselves in practice to enhance their grip on practice (Iedema and Merrick, 2008; Carroll and Mesman, 2018).

Now, the remainder of the chapter explains why VRE focuses on the *accomplishment of everyday practices*, outlining the difficulty and importance of looking at often taken-for-granted ways of working. We first delve into the literature that investigates the practice(s) of everyday work. Here, the concept 'habit' plays an important role, and 'exnovation' is introduced as describing the process of attending to the everyday unfolding of practices and the human habituations and capabilities that sustain those practices. Exnovation, we explain, depends on practitioners and patients being enabled to adopt different insider–outsider positions from which they become aware of different perspectives on everyday matters. Following that, we explain the role of video and feedback in producing these different positions and perspectives, and, in doing so, revealing the complexity of processes that are ordinarily taken for granted. We finish the chapter with a brief discussion about video footage as enabling viewers to see not just 'what was video-ed', but as in fact evoking a number of dimensions that normally remain buried in the hurly-burly of everyday care.

1.2 VISUALIZING THE INVISIBILITY OF EVERYDAY LIFE AND WORK

Increasingly, organizations, managers and professionals are realizing that work practices are in constant need of re-adjustment in order to respond effectively to constantly changing work contexts. To understand and improve work practice, however, we need to understand the way work is done. What is actually happening when people are at work? How do people accomplish their work? These kinds of questions are not easy to answer and have been a concern for the social sciences from their beginnings in the late 19th century. Since that time, and emerging from sociology, social psychology and management theory, approaches like Organizational Studies and Work Place Studies have revealed the complexity of our everyday work routines. Unravelling this complexity is at the heart of these endeavours' analytical foci, and this explains their affinity with VRE.

1.2.1 Studies of everyday work

Studies of everyday work take as their point of departure that *social interaction* among practitioners supported by various tools and technologies is the foundation for the accomplishment of work. These studies have a long tradition in describing how technologically supported social interaction produces and reproduces organizational forms, including the rules and procedures that inform these very same interactions. Unique in how they unpack this social accomplishment of work, Heath and Luff's work (2008) provides some critical guidance. First, they note, work is a situated activity. In other words, practical action is always situated in a specific context. For this reason, an analysis of work also requires an unpacking of the context in which the actions are produced.

Second, the situated nature of work implies that we should also attend to the contingent and variable ways in which activities are being accomplished. In other words, we need to attend to how participants respond to, reshape and reproduce the circumstances in which they accomplish their work. Their work-related activities are both context-sensitive and context-*renewing*. Hence, work is described as an 'emergent, interactional accomplishment of social action and activity' (Heath and Luff, 2008: 496).

Besides attending to the situational and dynamic character of social activity, Heath and Luff (2008) point out that 'unpacking' work practices requires attention to the social meanings attributed to the activities that are enacted, or the 'reasoning that inform[s] the concerted, collaborative accomplishment of practical action' (p. 496). This methodological advice thus suggests a detailed examination of care in terms of conversations, and the bodily and material conducts of those whose work we are interested in. This may involve a focus on the sequences by which interaction unfolds step by step, contextualized by the settings and cultures out of which actions are produced (Heath et al., 2004; Hindmarsh and Tutt, 2012).

No matter the investigative strategy (observations, recordings, interviews), in these sociological studies, work is considered as a collective and emergent product, and sensitive to the time and space in which it is produced. Viewing work as a situated activity explains the analytical focus on work practices or the 'modes of action and knowledge, emerging *in situ* from the dynamics of interactions' (Gherardi, 2006: 7).

Since the 1990s, many studies of work as situated activity emerged under the aegis of 'practice-based studies' (Schatzki et al., 2001). This 'practice turn' inspired us to see practices as primary, rather than (as traditional sociology had it) individual actors or sociological structures (Giddens, 1981). Practice theory saw social actors and social structures as produced and reproduced in everyday interaction (Schatzki, 1996). This perspective posited that 'the performance of practice' mobilized human and non-human actors, technologies, language, prior knowledge and background knowledge, tacit rules held by the community, and the historical, institutional and cultural contexts of work (Gherardi, 2012). This involved shifting our focus from work as made up of individuals engaged in more or less technologically extended activities, towards practice as a flow of activities that harness myriad phenomena, including human and non-human actors manifesting different levels of agency and path dependency (Callon and Latour, 1981).

The term 'practice' therefore is important, as it avoids long-standing dualisms separating people from social structures and cultural systems, as is typical of conventional dichotomies including agency/structure, human/non-human, knowledge/action and mind/body (Gherardi, 2012). The notion of practice is used to suggest that here-and-now human activity is always already produced by, and implicated in, iterating social and systemic phenomena, and vice versa.

The principal issue affecting the analysis of practice (and the *change* of practice) is to do with where we locate the origin of change (Nicolini, 2013). For some, practice may be the patterned ways of doing and being that are propagated and steered by (more or less fixed) social structures. Here, 'there is nothing new under the sun'. For example, and to a large extent, where we are born in society determines our social and economic achievements (Bourdieu, 1991). For others, practice needs to be performed into being every time anew, and no instantiation of practice is identical to another. Here, 'we never step into the same river twice'. Of course, both perspectives are valid. Practices are the outcome of 'an ongoing routinized and *recurrent accomplishment*' (Nicolini, 2013: 3), but their re-accomplishment is unlikely to remain identical over time. Seen through the lens of practice theory, understanding practices in order to change them therefore requires us to look 'behind' their durable features to see the processes that constitute and instantiate them.

1.2.2 Habits and practice

Another consideration is that practices are 'routine *bodily activities* made possible by the active contribution of an array of material resources' (Nicolini, 2013: 4). This bodily aspect of practice should not be seen as furnishing practice with 'a mere instrument', or the brawn that carries out instructions from the brain. Instead, we tend to speak about practice as realized through bodies and other material objects (Reckwitz, 2002), as well as through people's habits, assumptions, expectations and intentions (Dewey, 1922). Clearly, habits are central here. For Dewey (1922: 124), habits – and not conscious thought and strategic decision-making – are the primary means through which we engage with the world: 'Concrete habits do all the perceiving, recognizing, imagining, recalling, judging, conceiving and reasoning that is done'.

Habits tend to be well-settled bodily routines that only incur conscious attention when they come up against obstacles. On this view, practices are composed, to a greater or lesser extent, from habituated activities not requiring much conscious attention and mostly relying on 'muscle knowledge' (Shusterman, 2012). When thinking about practice change, therefore, we must consider actors' relationship to habits, their willingness to scrutinize habits and their inclination to render their habits changeable through reflexive practice, thereby rendering their habits 'intelligent' (Dewey, 1922).

Engaging the world through our habits further requires 'a way of *knowing* shared with others' (Nicolini, 2013: 5). That is, practising means sharing a background of inarticulate or 'tacit' knowledge and rules with others who co-participate in that practice. Wittgenstein (1953) referred to this by pointing out that practice can often only be justified by stating, 'This is simply what I do'. In other words, not everything we do is reasoned and explainable, but can be anchored in long-standing, tacit and unquestioned ways of doing and saying (Taylor, 1993).

Finally, practices realize interests in terms of what they are intended to accomplish. The term 'interests' keys in to the notions of *power* and power structures. Here, we focus on assumptions and conventions pertaining to who has the right to say what and when, and the right to do what and when. Power is ubiquitous: it is everywhere and continuous (Foucault, 1978). No practice operates without power, or without interests. Another way of putting this point is to say that practices have purposes, and purposes will serve some people and some causes better than others. That said, because power is ubiquitous, power is also never fixed. Particularly nowadays, social relationships and hierarchies are increasingly fluid, mainly thanks to intensifying levels of feedback (think of social media), the rising speed of information dissemination (the Internet) and rapid changes affecting resources and technologies (creating variabilities and unpredictabilities in what is valued and valuable).

Practice theory therefore promotes an image of what we do as steered, to greater or lesser extent, by phenomena that are not necessarily within our control: habits, sociocultural path dependencies, unquestioned background knowledge, practice-structuring technologies and, more recently, affects (Barnes, 2001; Blackman, 2013). But none of these are immune to reflexivity, or to enhanced intelligence, to use Dewey's (1922) terminology. VRE delves into 'what is' at the level of practice, which enables practitioners to attend to 'what is', and therefore renders human actors capable of perturbing the conditions that inform and sustain their work. This is what we refer to as the process of 'exnovation'.

1.3 EXNOVATION

In order to illuminate what goes into the accomplishment of health care, and to strengthen our grip on care complexity, VRE draws on the expertise of practitioners and other 'insiders'. Practitioners and insiders have a lived, practical knowledge of that complexity. We know however too that much of what practitioners do to accomplish their daily work activities involves unarticulated – and perhaps even unplanned yet effective – sets of actions. These actions may be as opaque to them and their colleagues, as they are to outsiders (and researchers). If we want to understand the way clinicians accomplish their everyday care work, we need to turn these everyday practices from taken-for-granted routines to activities of interest, or what Bruno Latour (2004) might term 'matters of concern'. Latour differentiated between how knowledge, things or practices can move from being 'matters of fact' – seen as unremarkable and taken for granted (such as a routine way of doing things) – to being 'matters of concern' – actions opened up to scrutiny in terms of how they are assembled and 'held together' in practice.

As noted previously, this includes attending to processes and dynamics that are taken as given, unquestioned or habituated. Above we set out Dewey's (1922) view that habits are the primary interface between human actors and their practical context and circumstances. In a sense, habits constitute the more or less 'hidden' competences of practitioners. We refer to habits as competencies because habits are the skilled outcome of actors' repeated interactions with their contexts (Dewey, 1922), even if habits run the risk of lapsing into blind, stubborn routines. The critical role of exnovation therefore is to illuminate and identify these already existing – but often overlooked or forgotten – competencies and resources. These competencies and resources are our habits, or our taken-as-given ways of doing, being and saying that structure much if not most of our behaviour. Enabling actors to reconnect with their habits on a conscious level in this way means enabling them to develop what Dewey calls 'intelligent habits' (Dewey, 1922). This process of reconnecting with our habits is what we term exnovation (De Wilde, 2000). Exnovation enables front-line actors to render their habits explicit, and render these habits intelligent by opening them up to revision and refinement in the light of their shifting contexts, information and circumstances.

As an aggregation of excavation (i.e. exposure to/of what is already there) and innovation, exnovation reanimates the implicit and hidden dimensions of practices (Mesman, 2011; Iedema et al., 2013). With its focus on the ways of doing and reasoning that are taken as given, and therefore less visible, exnovation acknowledges that these seemingly insignificant, informal and mundane actions act as crucial resources in the accomplishment of work practices. To exnovate these existing resources, we need to focus on how local actors enact ordinary and routine aspects of practice. However, even if we acknowledge the importance of reading practices 'from the inside', or 'from the point of view of the activity which is performed' (Gherardi, 2012: 161), this still leaves us with the question of how to overcome this opacity for both researchers and clinicians. VRE approaches this problem by multiplying perspectives on, experiences of and deliberations about what is going on.

1.4 THE INSIDER/OUTSIDER EFFECT

Experienced workers have an ability to conduct their work so skillfully that we sometimes say they have 'practical wisdom', or something that Aristotle referred to using the word *phronesis* (Flyvbjerg, 2001). But as workers, we also tend to embody a practical 'blindness' that prevents us from being aware of all aspects of our practice. Our world is often too familiar to fully come to our conscious attention, unless we come up against obstacles (Dewey, 1922). The shield of familiarity distances us from the many processes and actions we perform while doing all kinds of quite focused and demanding tasks. Thus, we may be typing while partaking in an interesting conversation. We may be listening to a radio programme while navigating through the traffic. We may be chatting with a patient while preparing his/her medications. For most of us, these taken-as-given dimensions of behaviour are fully functional, unless, of course, we find ourselves in situations where our typing is slowed by a different keyboard layout, or where our headphones distract us from critical traffic noises, or where the patient raises some critical concerns about their care – situations requiring us to pay attention to matters that were previously taken for granted.

Like most people, clinicians too are at times unable to 'see', much less discuss, the taken-for-granted – though crucial – aspects of their work. They may not have a language for talking about those aspects. Simply asking about these aspects using interviews, therefore, may be inadequate and insufficient for investigating or establishing what the work is that they do. To raise people's habits to awareness or to 'exnovate' these habits requires extra, and potentially confronting, questions. Here, an outsider's (more distant) perspective on people's practices (derived, say, through ethnographic observation and interviews) may also not suffice, because his/her perspective may be limited too. Indeed, outsiders' observations may highlight some things at the expense of others, and therefore offend practitioners as Becker and colleagues pointed out long ago, since outsiders'

> ... view of the world – abstract, relativistic, generalizing – necessarily deflates people's view of themselves and their organizations [because] something precious ... is treated as merely an instance of a class.
>
> (Becker et al., 1964: 273)

Using video, however, practitioners can re-view (repeatedly) and deliberate their actions. Such reviews and deliberations are most impactful when we bring together the 'lightly-cooked' footage of *in situ* practice with practitioners' insider knowledge (or their 'emic' knowledge; Pike, 1967: 43/4), with outsiders' perspectives (or what Pike refers to as 'etic' knowledge; Pike, 1967: 43/4). This convergence of footage and different perspectives serves to 'make the familiar strange'. 'Making the familiar strange' is a translation of Shklovskii's originally Russian expression *ostraneniye* (O'Toole and Shukman, 1977). Juxtaposing their own emic and others' etic perspectives helps professionals see familiar phenomena in a different light. Making things strange in this way enables professionals to reassess and re-appreciate their practice. From regarding their practice as an indisputable *matter of fact*, professionals may experience outsider perspectives as 'making things strange', and as turning what they do and who they are into *matters of concern*; that is, matters worthy of attention and deliberation, and perhaps change (Latour, 2004).

In the methodological literature, the advantages and disadvantages that attach to the roles of researcher-outsider and practitioner-insider have been hotly debated (Hammersley and Atkinson, 2010; Mannay, 2010). Some favour researchers as people who can 'objectively' observe what is going on, without being caught up in rules around what cannot be seen or said (Hammersley and Atkinson, 2010). Others favour the practitioner-insider role, as it is seen as having the best chance of shedding light on the hidden competencies and knowledge that inform practice (Bosk, 2003). Mesman (2007) and Hammersley and Atkinson (2010) point out, however, that both the insider and outsider positions are in essence 'mythical'. Both are narratives that claim to have a privileged access to a local world, and both therefore assume the existence of a stable and objective reality.

Mannay (2010, 2016) also acknowledges that both positions have shortcomings, but she further stresses that tensions and differences between the insider and outsider roles may be productive. That is the perspective taken here. We use the terms 'insider/outsider' and 'emic/etic' to underline the value of producing multiple perspectives on taken-as-given situations. These multiple perspectives may prompt insight, facilitate reflexivity for professionals, patients and researchers, and expand their collective understanding of how practices are accomplished and how they may be enhanced.

1.5 HOW VIDEO PROVIDES ACCESS TO COMPLEXITY

Much social scientific research that focuses on organizational practices demonstrates the complexity of these practices and of their accomplishment, even when the focus is on apparently simple tasks and day-to-day routines. Unpacking these practices includes paying attention to the details of work processes, such as mundane actions, verbal and other kinds of communication, the use of technologies and resources (including space and time), body movements and the knowledge and power structures that permeate and shape what goes on. The strands of social science specialized in capturing and analyzing these various facets of everyday work include (organizational) ethnography, conversation analysis, ethnomethodology, pragmatics (of organizations and professions) and symbolic interactionism, to name a few.

What these endeavours have in common is that they subject these complex social phenomena to descriptions and analyses that aim to extract general rules from them. For example, 'workplace studies', an off-shoot of conversation analysis pioneered by Christian Heath and colleagues, demonstrated that when doctors use computers during their consults, they have a tendency to turn away from their patients and focus on the computer screens for extended periods of the consult (Heath and Luff, 2000; Heath et al., 2000). Such patterns and regularities are informative and significant, and they may give practitioners much food for thought. By the same token, while these generalizations about human behaviour may be valid, their relevance for practitioners and patients may not be readily apparent. This happens when there is a disconnect between the ways in which these generalizations are derived and published, and the situated practices that legitimate and sustain such behaviours. For that reason, social scientific endeavours that unearth behavioural rules and regularities face a common challenge: How are such findings and conclusions made relevant to clinicians' and patients' *in situ* behaviour, understanding and interaction?

Progress towards strengthening the relevance of these micro-sociological phenomena for healthcare improvement may thus be hampered – ironically – by the disciplinary priorities that undergird these very social scientific research approaches. In fact, by viewing these micro-sociological phenomena through their disciplinary lens, these social science endeavours tend to construe social actors, their behaviours and the complex circumstances they inhabit as 'instances of a class' (to use Becker and colleagues' 1964 expression). This is how we expect science to operate: by privileging the 'gold standard' of generalization over specificity, these endeavours prioritize simplicity over complexity. But in a world where complexity is becoming more and more common and intense, general and simple or 'pre-cooked' answers no longer have the reach, applicability and efficacy they once may have had. Indeed, in such a world, we face the following dilemma: 'pre-cooked' answers and generalized solutions devised by 'experts elsewhere' no longer have a reliable purchase on the practical problems that people encounter in the here and now. Increasingly, novel ways forward have to be forged from within people's own unique circumstances (Sloterdijk, 2013).

For an alternative perspective on this dilemma, we look towards approaches that inhabit a rather different research paradigm – one that balances its own scientific and disciplinary ambitions against local stakeholders' aspirations, preferences and insights, and against sites' dynamics and instabilities. Approaches that spring to mind in this regard include action research, participative enquiry, transformative research and evaluation, and appreciative enquiry. These are approaches that position collaboration as central to (social) scientific enquiry. Collaboration with local stakeholders then is a critical strategy for addressing the dilemma posed by conventional 'grand' science not providing the full set of answers needed to key in to local tensions, problems, challenges and priorities. This alternative paradigm grants study subjects a prominent role in social science research and in organizational and practice improvement. Here, collaboration with professionals and patients becomes the means *par excellence* for engaging with complexity as it affects and challenges people in the here and now (Reason and Bradbury, 2008; Mertens, 2009; Iedema et al., 2013).

Only recently have health services research, patient safety and practice improvement begun to acknowledge that everyday phenomena, including human activity, are not just worthy of attention when things go wrong, but may offer a critical contribution to safety and improvement (Reason, 2008). The ways these everyday phenomena are currently framed however include complexity scientific abstractions (e.g. 'attractor', 'coevolution'), on the one hand (Braithwaite et al., 2017), and they are addressed using conventional scientific methods as the preferred means for deriving 'understanding' about these phenomena, on the other hand (Braithwaite, 2018). This literature's efforts are laudable for granting everyday phenomena an appropriate degree of attention. They remain wedded however to methodologies, solutions and role expectations that are hard pushed to meet the challenges posed by complexity.

The literature just reviewed may be forgiven for thinking that conventional methodologies, solutions and role expectations can shed light on complex phenomena. It is ultimately true that complexity is just another term for 'constrained diversity' (Wilden, 1987: 309). Diversity is constrained in more or less regular ways, and these regularities may be represented and illuminated in conventional ways. That said, complexity theory has made huge progress in recent years as it helps us make sense of the irreversibility and unpredictability of events. Complexity theory enables us to work with the uneasy relationship between (what we know about) the past and what (we can expect) will happen in the future (Prigogine, 1996). There is therefore more to tackling complexity than analyzing its past manifestations and its regularities, even if this is the route most commonly regarded as the most reliable and direct way to 'taming complexity' (Woods et al., 2007).

In our view, the problem runs more deeply than may be apparent from this literature's preference for conventional science. By positing a need for general *a priori* understandings of 'complexity dimensions' and by advocating standard methods as prime gateways into tackling complexity in general, this particular brand of healthcare improvement complexity science reveals its trajectory as 'proceeding from the "simple" to the "complex" (as 17th century "empiricists" and ideologists like John Locke (1632–1704) thought we should and could)' (Wilden, 1987: 314). This trajectory, paved with complexity scientific abstractions and tree-lined with conventional methods and analyses, essentially seeks refuge within a pre-complexity paradigm: 'the system ... is viewed as an object, and moreover as an object to be viewed or even "controlled" from an imaginary "outside" ' (Wilden, 1980: xxxviii).

The approach described in this book takes a very different trajectory. Instead of prioritizing that which is objective and generalizable (e.g. *a priori* understandings and analyses) as pre-conditions for how we deal with complexity, VRE engages with complexity as and when it happens. VRE does not require much special knowledge from participants or researchers. Hence, contrary to positing 'the simple' (the known, theory, results) as a pre-requisite for tackling 'the complex', VRE *harnesses complexity for dealing with complexity*. In Wilden's (1987: 314) terms, VRE moves 'from the complex to *the structures of complexity*, including their environments'. The complex is regarded as needing little to no pre-processing, and it is trusted to yield to participants' and researchers' sense-making. Tackling the complex as it manifests in real time illuminates and renders malleable its 'structures, including their environments' to those attending to it.

To access the complex, VRE mobilizes minimally processed technological means – video footage – for capturing and revisiting more or less complex events. Footage brings to the fore the moment-to-moment lived experiences, the habituations and practical knowledge of participants (professionals and patients) and the tangled realities of everyday care practices. As did Blake's (1863) 'grain of sand', a few seconds of footage may reveal a whole universe of complexity, particularly for those who are familiar with the sites, practices and processes captured in the footage. Footage makes possible more than the review of otherwise forgotten and taken-for-granted situations and events; it opens people up to the multi-layered, multi-dimensional and tenuous character of events and circumstances normally regarded as 'unremarkable'. In the following quote, Latour exemplifies this point:

> We say, without giving the matter too much thought, that we engage in 'face-to-face' interactions. Indeed we do, but the clothing that we are wearing comes from elsewhere and was manufactured a long time ago; the words we use were not formed for this occasion; the walls we have been leaning on were designed by an architect for a client, and constructed by workers-people who are absent today, although their action continues to make itself felt. The very person we are addressing is a product of a history that goes far beyond the framework of our relationship. If one attempted to draw a spatio-temporal map of what is present in the interaction, and to draw up a list of everyone who in one form or another were present, one would not sketch out a well-demarcated frame, but a convoluted … multiplicity of highly diverse dates, places and people.
>
> *(Latour, 1996: 231)*

Latour's insight becomes uniquely apparent when we view ourselves enacting work processes on a video screen. Participants reviewing situations and events captured on video recognize that seemingly unremarkable and insignificant work circumstances are in fact deeply intricate and complex. Witnessing every-day events and circumstances in this way may lead people to appreciate the complexity of common treatments, and the moment-to-moment accomplishment of patients' safety and quality of care. They may also appreciate the improvement potential of ordinary practices and processes, and the local manifestation of services and systems. In the section that follows, we expand on this 'hologrammatic effect' that viewing video footage may have on viewers.

More importantly still, witnessing complexity in how professionals and patients perform health care *in situ* may involve appreciating individuals' roles in and contributions to the unfolding of care on a range of levels. Indeed, recognizing complexity in everyday actions and circumstances may confirm people's sense of personal purpose and agency. The footage reveals that people are not just there to act out pre-scripted communication and pre-determined solutions, perhaps contrary to some extent to the felt experience of many working in health care. People realize they are far from automatons negotiating predictable situations, activities and processes. On the contrary, they are there to attend to and navigate through an infinite array of complex events. People's sense of purpose for being at work and being valued at work is therefore strengthened: the significance of their agency amidst complexity is thrown into stark relief against the backdrop of static rules, knowledges and routines that contextualize how they enact care.

The foregoing may now be distilled into a single proposition: Complexity is not a problem to be solved but an opportunity that necessitates and motivates people to acknowledge and realize their responsibility and agency. Their sense of responsibility and agency arises from the realization that *in situ* care *cannot* be fully managed and determined on the basis of simple rules and solutions handed down from above or borrowed from elsewhere: how care unfolds in the 'here and now' is inevitably conditional on how individuals navigate and negotiate its complex unfolding.

Latour's quote, mentioned previously, thus helps expand our vision out from the 'here and now' into a past and a future 'there and then'. It highlights that, in essence, we are all implicated in numerous complex circumstances, events and systems. We can take this further, and say that our sense that things are simple and regular is in fact no more than a product of a series of decisions we make about where to draw boundaries around who we are, what we do and what we pay attention to. Recognizing this is the first step towards acknowledging our significance as actors in these processes, and potentially towards intervening in how complexities unfold in our life and work.

That said, we also need to acknowledge that we may not always recognize and effectively deal with the complexities we encounter. We tend to focus on the issues that matter *now* and may ignore ones that we assume can be taken as given, or treated as mere *context*. Consider this by way of example: to participate in sterile procedures in the neonatal unit, we need to be able to key in to the minute gestures, postures, communication and actions that contribute to the achievement of this sterility (Mesman, 2009). Participating in this practice is contingent on taking account of other people's moves, the onset and completion of actions and the role divisions that contribute to the accomplishment of such work, among many other things (Mesman, 2009). Over time, practitioners come to embody these sensitivities and act on them without needing to fully render them conscious and explicit (Collins and Evans, 2002). They have become *background* to other activities, which are now central and focal.

The term 'background' is important here. For Taylor (1993), 'background' refers to everything in our context(s) that makes it possible for us to function in everyday life. This context may embody simple things like knowing how to tie our laces without thinking too much about it. It may also include our experience of being able to 'read' a patient and use our gut feelings to work out what to do next. The background is where we store all that which we take as given. In Taylor's sense, the background thus encompasses our cultural customs and social routines, as well as their personal equivalent: our habits.

As referred to earlier, our habits inhabit an intermediate space between automatic reflex (e.g. withdrawing our hand from a burning hot radiator) and reasoned, conscious action. Habits encompass a domain of purposive human conduct where activity and decision-making have stabilized to such a degree that people may spend limited time thinking about what they do. Activity has been allowed to become 'automatic'. In the healthcare research literature, habits tend to be described as products or symptoms of culture. In that guise, they may act as a source of inertia or even resistance, or be a mere manifestation of our human cognitive shortcomings.

In contrast, Dewey (1922) saw habits as a form of *intelligence*. He regarded habits as intelligent, not just because they mediate between humans and their environments, creating a behavioural economy. Dewey went further in that he saw habits as capable of being rendered *more* intelligent by being brought (back) into consciousness, rendering them amenable to being re-evaluated and reshaped. Becoming aware of our habits, he argued, gives us a special grip on what tends otherwise to remain taken-as-given in the background. The following quote is from Shusterman, a keen Dewey scholar, who comments on this issue:

> Your habitual way of walking depends not only on your particular physical structure (itself partly shaped by habits of nutrition and movement that shape muscle and eventually even the bone) but also on the surfaces on which you walk, the shoes you walk in, the exemplars of walking you witness and attune yourself to, and the situational purposes that frame your customary gait (rushing to work through crowded streets versus leisurely strolling barefoot on the sand). Habits of thought must likewise incorporate features of the environment that are necessary or worthwhile to think about and address through action. Moreover, since habits are formed over time, they also embody environmental histories and thus can persist even when the original conditions are no longer present … .
>
> *(Shusterman, 2008: 190)*

With the advent of video, we have a unique resource for making our habits accessible to ourselves, thereby rendering them more intelligent. Video-facilitated observation engages participants in paying attention to ordinary, taken-as-given (inter)actions. Doing so creates 'an opportunity to open up for *dwelling* on the minute details of performance, and through which practices become realized – something that would be impossible to do during face-to-face interaction' (Martens, 2012: 47). Video recordings are powerful because they offer an alternative take on and repeatable view of the unfolding activity in the here and now. This is what makes video unique: it brings us a little closer to infinitely complex phenomena that ordinarily remain in (or are relegated to) 'the background': all the circumstances, actions, resources and causes that come together in our present, the living here and now.

By capturing and replaying (some of) these phenomena, video footage is able to demonstrate, not just for researchers but also for the people portrayed in it, the importance of body conduct, gestural work, tool use and interactive technologies for the conduct of relationships and for the enactment of care work (Hindmarsh and Tutt, 2012). Video recordings afford the possibility to zoom in, rewind, play back, share, slow down, speed up, annotate and analyze everyday actions and activities in ways never before possible (Hindmarsh and Tutt, 2012). These affordances are capitalized on in the insightful work by Christian Heath and colleagues. In one article, for example, they describe all the actions involved in a 15-s shot of a moment of everyday work in an anaesthetic room in a hospital (Heath et al., 2010: 6).

By visualizing behavioural rhythms, duration and real-time production of work in this way, video footage enables us to examine the spatial–temporal ordering of practices. Where numerical data reduces contextual information and complexity in order to see overarching patterns and trends, video *foregrounds* complex contextual details and circumstances. But since our culture sets great store by simplicity, the criticality and functionality of complexity is rarely acknowledged. Complexity has been framed as a problem to be understood, and then 'tamed'. And yet, such thinking ignores the fact that complexity embodies movement and change, and movement and change invite attention and participation. As such, complexity creates subtle anchor points for recognition, engagement, connection, creativity and memory. Unless life veers off into chaos, leaving us overwhelmed, confused, uncertain and alone, complexity can be enabling, moving and engaging.

But even if life seems chaotic to us, replaying and reviewing such complex events on video offers us opportunities to share and mitigate our confusion and uncertainty. Doing so may alert us to previously unnoticed regularities and other reassuring aspects of reality. As relatively unprocessed or 'under-cooked' portrayal of what went on, video edges close to the original density and intensity of what happens. As under-cooked record, video affords and invites multiple experiences, interpretations and perspectives, and leaves room for ambiguity and disagreement. For instance, did we seriously mean to conduct our ambulance-to-emergency handover in this busy corridor with no space to move in between no fewer than *four* patients in their beds and too much noise to properly hear one another (Figure 1.1)?

Or, did we intend to interrupt this clinical handover by walking straight through the clinical team meeting and draw the attention of one of the doctors without respecting and paying attention to what was being discussed (Figure 1.2; see the arrow indicating someone's outstretched arm trying to get the taller

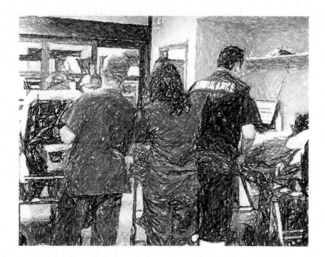

Figure 1.1 Ambulance to ED handover.

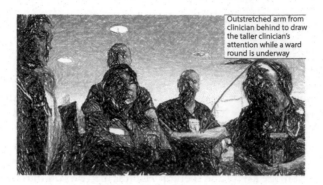

Figure 1.2 Ward round handover interrupted.

clinician's attention)? Did the clinical team stop the handover during the interruption in the interest of everyone staying informed, or did the team continue as if the interruption did not happen?

We can use these examples too to explain why video footage is inevitably *polysemic*, that is, open to multiple meanings and interpretations. We may be used to the noise, the lack of space and the interruptions, and we may feel confident that our work is safe and effective. In contrast, others may be bewildered by the noise and the constant movements, and see that significant things are missed or routinely ignored, or that people's routines just do not make sense: they are inefficient, perhaps even dangerous. Watching themselves perform taken-as-given activities, people may see things of which they were not previously conscious: did we as emergency department triage staff really behave so dismissively towards the ambulance paramedics? Have we resigned ourselves to how emergency clinicians ignore our ambulance handovers (Iedema et al., 2012)?

Of course, this is not to say that our interpretation of what we see in video footage may never be problematic. Rose (2016) explains how interpretations are intertwined with the institutional and ideological order(s) in which those who watch the video are ensconced. In other words, the array of meanings attributed to footage is likely to be bounded by the backgrounds (i.e. the social practices, institutions and relations) from within which the footage is produced, viewed and interpreted. This renders video 'polysemic, ambiguous and multi-modal' (Mannay, 2016: 66) in that it captures a wealth of gestures, movements, talk and all kinds of other ways in which people communicate and work together. This multiplicity invites multiple perspectives (not always in agreement) as to what it is about, what its function is or how justified and appropriate it is.

This challenge is not eased by the fact that thanks to technological developments, video enables us to capture, store and replay the 'here and now' with greater speed and intensity. We can now portray what goes on using not just 2D video, but also 3D video that captures 360° of what goes on around the camera. This yields a lot of information, allowing a level of access, detail, flexibility and scrutiny never experienced before, and likely to affect our consciousness of ordinary interaction (Thrift, 2005). In all, video opens up our taken-for-granted reality/realities revealing its/their complex unfolding and rich textures.

Finally, we should not think that video is just about 'seeing' (Grasseni, 2007). The incorrectness of this assumption will become clear as we move on, not least when we discuss how video footage embodies a very prominent 'felt' or *affective* dimension. This manifests in people who view footage of themselves and become conscious of how they enact their relationships with others, of the feelings they embody towards them and of how such feelings, upon reflection, may add a very special dimension to practice that they were not aware of, or may seem entirely inappropriate and out of place.

The way in which video footage foregrounds affect can be quite pronounced. In one meeting, senior doctors commented on how surprised they were to see themselves intimidate junior doctors during a ward round (Carroll et al., 2008). Aileen Collier's work involved showing clinicians who had cared for patients who were now dying, the footage of these patients' pre-death experiences and circumstances: declared 'futile', shunted away from the main corridors of care, sometimes into windowless rooms with paint falling off the walls, they were waiting to die. The footage had an indelible affective impact on the clinicians involved (Collier, 2013). We return to the affective dimension of video feedback in later chapters.

1.6 VIDEO FOOTAGE AS 'HOLOGRAM'

In saying that video embodies a *polysemy*, we seek to emphasize its three unique affordances.

First, besides making it possible to see again, video footage makes it possible for people to *hear* again, to *feel* again and to *think, question* and *remember* again. Video has an ontological impact, thanks to being able to affect people in all these ways (MacDougall, 2006).

Second, the term 'polysemy' underscores the variety of perspectives and interpretations that are likely to come to light when we are made aware of the complexity of the taken-for-granted, the background. We witness our own practice and behaviour and come to realize we have different understandings and knowledge about what goes on. The patina of social alignment instead now appears as a cracked, multi-layered and multi-coloured varnish shot through with differing assumptions and rationales (Iedema et al., 2018). As a result, reviewing video footage may surprise people, revealing their practices and relationships as somewhat less coordinated, cohesive and logical than pre-supposed.

Third, the term 'polysemy' applies to video footage on yet another level, in that it may reveal multiple facets of everyday activity. Thus, a few seconds of video footage may enable people to remember circumstances further into the past, as well as what happened going into the future. In essence, this is because video footage takes on the appearance of a *hologram* for its viewers. Here, the word 'hologram' is used to describe a multi-layered sensorium that is much more than a simple picture or reflection of 'what happened' (Iedema et al., 2013).

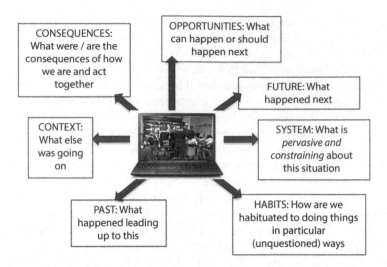

Figure 1.3 The hologrammatic potential of video footage.

This multi-layered or hologrammatic character of video footage can be depicted and described as follows: Figure 1.3 portrays a screen with footage linked to arrows that point in different directions. The different arrows' directions are labelled 'past', 'future', 'context', 'system', 'habits', 'consequences' and 'opportunities'. These arrows go towards fleshing out the various affordances of video footage for those viewing it.

Thus, upon reviewing the footage, we have found that participants can see back into the past before the footage was shot. They also see into the future beyond the end point of the footage. They can further 'see' or sense the context in which the videoed activities took place. They may become aware of the pervasive or systemic aspects of what is going on, and of their own habits and their role in perpetuating that which is portrayed on the screen. They can often see the consequences of this confluence of context, system and habits, and they may be able to see the opportunities that are embedded in what is going on – opportunities as simple and logical as changing the time and place of handover (Carroll et al., 2008; Iedema, 2009), formalizing how they share information with colleagues (Iedema et al., 2012) or changing how they engage with patients at the ends of their lives and how they communicate with patients about healthcare-associated infections (Collier and Wyer, 2016). In short, watching footage should not be mistaken to involve 'seeing only what is on the screen'. On the contrary, viewing video footage brings much, much more to life for those involved.

By the same token, we must not assume that images provide us a well-washed and fully transparent window onto the world (Rose, 2016). It may be helpful here to distinguish between vision and visuality. Vision refers to our physiological ability of seeing. Visuality, on the other hand, refers to how vision is constructed: 'how we see, how we are able, allowed, or made to see, and how we see this seeing and the unseen therein' (Foster, 1988: p. ix, as cited in Rose, 2016: 3). Vision is what is on the screen. Visuality is what we – potentially *hologrammatically* – make of what we see on the screen.

This vision–visuality distinction is also helpful for considering what we fail to see. Inevitably, footage portrays some people, actions and things, while absenting others. The hologrammatic character of video is posited here as a way of underscoring that what is not shown or seen can be as important as what is shown and seen. Different people may see different things, and they may infer different things from what is shown (Hirshauer, 2006). Through discussing what is shown (vision) and what is seen (visuality), we may be able to retrieve events and experiences that are critical for understanding how people see practice as unfolding and why practice unfolds as it does. Indeed, without such discussion, we fail to capitalize on the unique affordance of video as providing an entry point into our taken-as-given backgrounds: the realm of unquestioned habits.

We therefore should not regard footage simply as 'showing' the world (Pink, 2007). Instead, when we create and watch footage, we are *co-constructing* (and making tangible) particular entry points into seeing, apprehending and acting on the world. Our entry points are necessarily a matter of reflexivity, not only for participants but also for researchers who reflect on who holds the camera, who makes decisions about what is videoed, who is included in the view, for how long and from which angles. Reflexivity continues into the decisions that are made about what footage is chosen to be shown, who is invited to view and comment on the footage during reflexive sessions and how these sessions are facilitated. These are all tactical decisions applied to the context of interest, determining what is 'found' and what is 'relevant'.

1.7 CONCLUSION

This chapter has sketched out some of the basic principles, theories and methodological considerations that underpin VRE. Video footage has been shown to provide access to everyday complexity. VRE enables participants to be alerted to the aspects of everyday complexity that they have learned to forget. The unique affordance of video is that it is polysemic: it engages participants with what happened in different registers, it opens up for participants different perspectives and interpretations and it enables participants to project what they see into unseen but experienced or suspected pasts and futures. In what follows, we delve more deeply into video as a practical resource for engaging with and intervening in complex care circumstances.

REFERENCES

Barnes B. (2001) Practice as collective action. In: Schatzki T, Knorr-Cetina K, and von Savigny E (eds) *The Practice Turn in Contemporary Theory.* London: Routledge, 17–28.

Becker HS, Geer B, Hughes EC, et al. (1964) *Boys in White: Student Culture in Medical School.* New Brunswick: Transaction Publishers.

Blackman L. (2013) Habit and affect: Revitalizing a forgotten history. *Body and Society* 19: 186–216.

Blake W. (1863) Auguries of Innocence. Retrieved from: https://www.poetryfoundation.org/poems/43650/auguries-of-innocence

Bleakley A. (1999) From reflexive practice to holistic reflexivity. *Studies in Higher Education* 24: 315–330.

Bosk C. (2003) *Forgive and Remember: Managing Medical Failure*. Chicago, IL and London: University of Chicago Press.

Bourdieu P. (1991) *Language & Symbolic Power*. Cambridge, MA: University of Harvard.

Braithwaite J. (2018) Changing how we think about healthcare improvement. *British Medical Journal*. doi:10.1136/bmj.k2014.

Braithwaite J, Churucca K, Ellis LA, et al. (2017) *Complexity Science in Health Care: Aspirations, Approaches, Applications and Accomplishments*. Sydney: Australian Institute of Health Innovation, Macquarie University.

Callon M and Latour B. (1981) Unscrewing the big Leviathan: How actors macro-structure reality and how sociologists help them to do so. In: Knorr-Cetina K and Cicourel AV (eds) *Advances in Social Theory and Methodology: Toward an Integration of Micro- and Macro-Sociologies*. Boston, MA: Routledge & Kegan Paul, 277–303.

Carroll K, Iedema R and Kerridge R. (2008) Reshaping ICU ward round practices using video reflexive ethnography. *Qualitative Health Research* 18: 380–390.

Carroll K and Mesman J. (2018) Multiple researcher roles in video-reflexive ethnography. *Qualitative Health Research* 28: 1145–1156.

Collier A. (2013) Deleuzians of Patient Safety: A Video Reflexive Ethnography of End-of-Life Care. PhD Thesis. Sydney: Faculty of Arts and Social Sciences, University of Technology.

Collier A and Wyer M. (2016) Researching reflexively with patients and families: Two studies using video-reflexive ethnography to collaborate with patients and families in patient safety research. *Qualitative Health Research* 26: 979–993.

Collins H and Evans R. (2002) The third wave of science studies: Studies of expertise and experience. *Social Studies of Science* 32: 235–296.

Davidoff F. (2002) Shame: The elephant in the room. *Quality and Safety in Health Care* 11: 2–3.

De Wilde R. (2000) Innovating Innovation: A contribution to the philosophy of the future. *Paper Read at the Policy Agendas for Sustainable Technological Innovation Conference*, London.

Dewey J. (1922) *Human Nature and Conduct: An Introduction to Social Psychology*. New York: H. Holt & Company.

Edmondson A. (1999) Psychological safety and learning behavior in work teams. *Administrative Science Quarterly* 44: 350–383.

Edmondson A. (2002) Managing the risk of learning: Psychological safety in work teams. In: West M (ed) *International Handbook of Organizational Teamwork*. London: Blackwell, 255–275.

Flyvbjerg B. (2001) *Making Social Science Matter: Why Social Science Fails and How It Can Succeed Again.* Cambridge: Cambridge University Press.

Foster H. (1988) Preface. In Foster H (ed) *Vision and Visuality.* Seattle: Bay Press. ix–xiv.

Foucault M. (1978) *The History of Sexuality (Volume I).* Harmondsworth: Penguin.

Gherardi S. (2006) *Organizational Knowledge: The Texture of Workplace Learning.* Oxford: Blackwell.

Gherardi S. (2012) *How to Conduct a Practice-Based Study: Problems and Methods.* Cheltenham: Edward Elgar.

Giddens A. (1981) Agency, institution, and time-space analysis. In: Knorr-Cetina K and Cicourel AV (eds) *Advances in Social Theory and Methodology: Toward an Integration of Macro- and Micro-Sociologies.* Boston, MA: Routledge & Kegan Paul, 161–174.

Goodyear-Smith F, Jackson C and Greenhalgh T. (2015) Co-design and implementation research: Challenges and solutions for ethics committees. *BMC Medical Ethics* 16: 78.

Grasseni C. (2007) *Killed Visions: Between Apprenticeship and Standards.* Oxford: Berghahn.

Hammersley M and Atkinson P. (2010) *Ethnography: Principles in Practice.* London: Routledge.

Heath C, Hindmarsh J and Luff P. (2010) *Video in Qualitative Research: Analysing Social Interaction in Everyday Life.* Los Angeles, CA: Sage.

Heath C, Knoblauch H and Luff P. (2000) Technology and social interaction: The emergence of 'workplace studies'. *The British Journal of Sociology* 51: 299–320.

Heath C and Luff P. (2000) Documents and professional practice: 'Bad' organisational reasons for 'good' clinical records. In: Heath C and Luff P (eds) *Technology in Action.* Cambridge: Cambridge University Press, 31–60.

Heath C and Luff P. (2008) Video and the analysis of work and interaction. In: Alasuutari P, Bickman L and Brannen J (eds) *The Sage Handbook of Social Research Methods.* Los Angeles, CA: Sage, 493–505.

Heath C, Luff P and Knoblauch H. (2004) Tools, technologies and organizational interaction: The emergence of 'workplace studies'. In: Grant D, Hardy C and Oswick C, et al. (eds) *The Sage Handbook of Organizational Discourse.* London: Sage, 337–375.

Hindmarsh J and Tutt D. (2012) Video in analytic practice. In: Pink S (ed) *Advances in Visual Methodology.* London: Sage, 57–73.

Hirshauer S. (2006) Puttings things into words. Ethnographic description and the silence of the social. *Human Studies* 2: 413–441.

Iedema R, Ball C, Daly B, et al. (2012) Design and trial of a new ambulance-to-emergency department handover protocol: 'IMIST-AMBO'. *BMJ Quality & Safety* 21: 627–633.

Iedema R, Jorm C, Hooker C, et al. (2018) To follow a rule? On frontline clinicians' understandings and embodiments of hospital-acquired infection prevention and control rules. Health. doi:10.1177/1363459318785677.

Iedema R and Merrick E. (2008) *HELiCS: Handover – Enabling Learning in Communication for Safety: A Handover Improvement Kit.* Sydney: Australian Commission on Safety & Quality in Health Care.

Iedema R, Merrick E, Rajbhandari D, et al. (2009) Viewing the taken-for-granted from under a different aspect: A video-based method in pursuit of patient safety. *International Journal for Multiple Research Approaches* 3: 290–301.

Iedema R, Mesman J, Carroll K. (2013) *Visualising Health Care Improvement: Innovation from Within.* Oxford: Radcliffe.

Jackson AY and Mazzei LA. (2012) *Thinking with Theory in Qualitative Research: Viewing Data across Multiple Perspectives.* Abingdon: Routledge.

Lather P. (2013) Methodology-21: What do we do in the afterward? *International Journal of Qualitative Studies in Education* 26: 634–645.

Latour B. (1996) On interobjectivity. *Mind, Culture and Activity* 3: 228–245.

Latour B. (2004) Why has critique run out of steam? From matters of fact to matters of concern. *Critical Enquiry* 30: 225–248.

MacDougall D. (2006) *The Corporeal Image: Film, Ethnography and the Senses.* Princeton, NJ: Princeton University Press.

Mannay D. (2010) Making the familiar strange: Can visual research methods render the familiar setting more perceptible? *Qualitative Research* 10: 91–111.

Mannay D. (2016) *Visual, Narrative and Creative Research Methods: Application, Reflection and Ethics.* Abingdon: Routledge.

Martens L. (2012) The politics and practices of looking: CCTV video and domestic kitchen practices. In: Pink S (ed) *Advances in Visual Methodology.* London: Sage, 39–56.

Mertens DM. (2009) *Transformative Research and Evaluation.* New York: Guildford Press.

Mesman J. (2007) Disturbing observations as a basis for collaborative research. *Science as Culture* 16: 281–295.

Mesman J. (2009) The geography of patient safety: A topical analysis of sterility. *Social Science & Medicine* 69: 705–1712.

Mesman J. (2011) Resources of strength: An exnovation of hidden competences to preserve patient safety. In: Rowley E and Waring J (eds) *A Sociocultural Perspective on Patient Safety.* Farnham: Ashgate, 71–92.

Nicolini D. (2013) *Practice Theory, Work, and Organization: An Introduction.* Oxford: Oxford University Press.

O'Toole M and Shukman A. (1977) A contextual glossary of formalist critical terminology. In: O'Toole M and Shukman A (eds) *Russian Poetics in Translation (Volume 4).* Oxford: Holdan Books, 1–45.

Pike K. (1967) *Language in Relation to a Unified Theory of the Structure of Human Behaviour.* The Hague: Mouton & Co.

Pink S. (2007) *Doing Visual Ethnography: Images, Media and Representation in Research.* London: Sage.

Prigogine I. (1996) *The End of Certainty: Time, Chaos and the New Laws of Nature*. New York: The Free Press.

Reason J. (2008) *The Human Contribution: Unsafe Acts, Accidents and Heroic Recoveries*. Farnham: Ashgate.

Reason P and Bradbury H. (2008) *The Sage Handbook of Action Research: Participative Inquiry and Practice*. London: Sage.

Reckwitz A. (2002) Toward a theory of social practices: A development in culturalist theorizing. *European Journal of Social Theory* 5: 243–263.

Rose G. (2016) *Visual Methodologies: An Introduction to Researching with Visual Materials*. Los Angeles, CA: Sage.

Schatzki T. (1996) *Social Practices: A Wittgensteinian Approach to Human Activity and the Social*. Cambridge: Cambridge University Press.

Schatzki T, Knorr-Cetina K and Savigny E. (2001) *The Practice Turn in Contemporary Theory*. London/New York: Routledge.

Shusterman R. (2008) *Body Consciousness: A Philosophy of Mindfulness and Somaesthetics*. Cambridge: Cambridge University Press.

Shusterman R. (2012) *Thinking through the Body: Essays in Somasthetics*. Cambridge: Cambridge University Press.

Sloterdijk P. (2013) *You Must Change Your Life*. Cambridge: Polity Press.

Taylor C. (1993) To follow a rule …. In: Calhoun C, LiPuma E and Postone M (eds) *Bourdieu: Critical Perspectives*. Cambridge: Polity Press, 45–60.

Thrift N. (2005) From born to made: Technology, biology and space. *Transactions of the Institute of British Geographers* 30: 463–476.

Wilden A. (1980) *System and Structure: Essays in Communication and Exchange*. London: Tavistock.

Wilden A. (1987) *The Rules Are No Game: The Strategy of Communication*. London: Routledge & Kegan Paul.

Wittgenstein L. (1953) *Philosophical Investigations*. Oxford: Blackwell.

Woods DD, Patterson ES and Cook RI. (2007) Behind human error: Taming complexity to improve patient safety. In: Carayon P (ed) *Handbook of Human Factors and Ergonomics in Health Care and Patient Safety*. Mahwah, NJ: Lawrence Erlbaum Associates, 459–476.

2

Preparing for fieldwork and collaborative data construction

2.1 INTRODUCTION

In this and subsequent chapters, we will equip you with the necessary tools, processual knowledge and tips to fund, plan and commence video-reflexive ethnography (VRE) in a healthcare setting. Using direct experience as the basis of our case studies, in this chapter we will elaborate the following topics: building relationships with key stakeholders (which includes negotiating field access, reassuring clinical participants about the use of video and setting the research agenda with clinical partners), attracting research funding, submitting an application to Human Research Ethics Committees (HRECs)/ Institutional Review Boards (IRBs), and visual and legal ethics including data retention.

2.2 PUTTING TOGETHER RESEARCH TEAMS FOR A VRE PROJECT

There are several considerations when putting together a VRE project team. The team you put together will, like any research team, be defined by the context and nature of the project and the skills and experience required within the team. While your proposal identifies clear role allocations and team rationales, in practice people's roles may be much less strictly defined than in conventional research studies. The organic unfolding of VRE research may result in people's roles and contributions developing in unexpected directions. For this reason, the team will need to include people who are flexible and not overly protective of their disciplinary training and background. VRE engages with complex phenomena, and this engagement itself is therefore unlikely to be simple and linear.

2.3 BUILDING RELATIONSHIPS WITH KEY STAKEHOLDERS AND DESIGNING YOUR STUDY OR PROJECT

In our experience, setting up a VRE project requires time and patience and much tenacity. You can never start talking too early with the people you are hoping to involve in your study. Try to draw on and build from existing relationships and partnerships. If you are embarking on VRE for the first time, take it slowly. For example, plan to start in a single setting, and choose one where you and your work are likely to be known or welcomed. Avoid sites where there are difficult issues, conflicts or disquiet among staff. It only takes one senior clinician's single objection to put a halt to an entire project. Generating interest and building trust take time, and you will need to be prepared to present and re-present the research to multiple parties and in different ways. It is helpful to allow for this 'legwork' in your budget and planning.

An example may be helpful at this point. In one of our studies, endorsement of the research by the Area Medical Director paved the way to access three acute hospital sites. We wrote to all relevant General Managers and Directors of Nursing at these sites to explain the project and reassure them that filming would only occur in close collaboration with clinical staff on the ground. We also gave these senior managers the opportunity to meet face-to-face with us in order to discuss the project in greater depth. We soon realized that speaking with people once might not be sufficient, and we needed to request access to a variety of meetings and gatherings to explain the approach and the principles underpinning it, especially to our potential participants at the front-line. Encountering the same people a number of times and explaining the project to different audiences gave people several opportunities to become comfortable with us as individuals and as a team, ask questions, think through the implications of what was on offer, and benefit from hearing colleagues express their thoughts and reservations, as well as being 'nudged along' by colleagues' interest in what was proposed, their possible previous experience with it and their approval.

Given that so much depends on your presentations to different clinician and manager audiences, you need to think carefully about how to pitch the project or study. It is important to recognize that different audiences may require different strategies and different pitches. In the following table, we provide a couple of examples of 'elevator' pitches: descriptions you can use to persuade people if all you have is 30s of their attention (see Table 2.1).

Senior executive level people are likely to have different questions, agendas and concerns compared to front-line clinicians. Senior staff may be persuaded to lend their support once they understand that this research promotes the involvement of front-line clinicians in and their learning about not just solving local, everyday problems, but also creating opportunities for realizing new policies and guidelines. Importantly, senior staff needs to be reassured that appropriate (legal and ethical) governance principles will apply to how the project deals with care challenges, incidents and conflicts.

Table 2.1 Examples of pitches

Pitch for senior management	VRE provides a way of connecting front-line staff to the edicts of health service reform and practice improvement. When new guidelines and policies are issued, front-line staff may be too busy and preoccupied to figure out how to accommodate the new rules in what they do. Seeing themselves providing care to patients gives staff opportunities for seeing where and how change can occur. This approach further involves them in making changes relevant to them and their patients, and this supports their well-being. VRE is governed by very specific principles ensuring full confidentiality of those involved and safe storage of data. For these and related reasons, we have received the support from some of the largest and most highly regarded healthcare services in the world, including Royal Prince Alfred Hospital in Sydney, Melbourne Health, the Mayo Clinic in Rochester (USA), Maastricht University Hospital and the University Medical Center Utrecht in the Netherlands.
Pitch for front-line staff	We know there are constant demands made on you to improve and change your practices. VRE gives you control over how you work and what you change, opening up your everyday work for your own scrutiny. For example, think of a time when you may have observed yourself on video: serving at tennis, delivering a speech at a wedding or conducting a patient consult. Such feedback moments are engraved in people's memories because they reveal so much for them, giving them the power to adjust the aspects of their behaviour of which they had previously not been aware. We know that some people are uncomfortable with being videoed, but VRE puts you in the driver's seat when it comes to deciding what to video, what to play back, what to critique and what to treasure in how you work. We also make sure that others will not see any footage of you without your express permission. Researchers have found that VRE gives participants new insights into their ways of working, to identify opportunities for change and to devise for themselves meaningful strategies that work for your particular context. It is very similar to what high-achieving athletes and sports teams do to improve their practices.

Front-line professionals are more likely to be interested in the practical dynamics of VRE, the demands on their time, the specifics of how confidentiality is maintained, and the legal and ethical dimensions that attach to the production and use of video footage. That said, professionals may have been involved in television programmes and have been subjected to filming by large film crews. They may even have seen themselves in reality TV programmes in unexpected ways. The most persuasive argument for front-line professionals we find is the one that states that musicians, singers, athletes and high-achieving sports people make regular use of video to enhance their performances. Indeed, sports matches now involve coaches regularly sending video clips of games down to players who cycle in and out of the field with advice to watch the clips, reflect on their performance, and learn, *in situ* and in real time.

Let us also elaborate on some of the more challenging aspects of persuading people to be videoed. One central challenge relates to project stakeholders' expectations about and perspectives on the ultimate point and purpose of the project, on the reasons underpinning the approach used, and on how (visual) data is expected to be collected, analysed and disseminated (Cox et al., 2014). Even though roles are likely to evolve over the course of the project, Cox and colleagues suggest it is important to give thought to who will commit to what kinds of roles and who is expected to own footage and dissemination products, particularly when there are multiple stakeholders involved in a project. It is also important to negotiate in advance what artefacts are likely to arise from the research and how these are to be used (Cox et al., 2014).

Will ownership of visual data be shared for example? Will outputs be shared? If the research involves partner organizations, do you need to have a written agreement early in the project as to where visual outputs will be stored and who will be responsible for them in the longer term according to institutional and legal regulations? Will participants and/or co-researchers see or perhaps even retain a copy of the footage? Who will decide how visual outputs are represented in the context of the wider research or project, and will everyone involved have a say in this regard?

Front-line clinicians (and their managers) may also be concerned about individuals or teams being filmed doing the wrong thing, or doing things the wrong way. Showing them videoed examples of real care practice may help persuade them of the richness of real-time video footage and the myriad things professionals can learn from it. This is by no means to deny the occurrence of clinical incidents, of course, nor to deny the possibility of you capturing an incident on video. The advantage of a video is that the hologrammatic effect of video-reflexivity allows us to bring factors to light that go beyond a specific individual's actions and decisions. Rather than showing an individual's culpability, footage of clinical care is more likely to foreground the pervasiveness of multiple factors. Paradoxically, video may capture a single person's activity, but in doing so, it illuminates much more than individual cognition and action, foregrounding the habitual, circumstantial, social, systemic and otherwise pervasive features of activity. It shows individuals' reasoning and intention to be entangled with numerous extra- and non-individual factors.

To finish this part of the discussion, we should mention that in our 18 years of using video in acute care settings, we once videoed two junior doctors debating over what to do while their patient started to arrest in the bed next to them. A senior doctor had to run towards them and intervene to save the patient.

But rather than incriminating the junior doctors, the footage, when reviewed, revealed they were all acting at the optimum of their ability and knowledge. Another time, we videoed two intensive care clinicians handing over information that did not apply to the patient in front of them. When we asked him what to do with the clip that captured this incorrect handover, the Director of the Intensive Care Unit (who was one of the people handing over) asked if he could use the clip of this interaction at international conferences to argue that reflecting on *in situ* practice using footage of real-time care is critical to learning about how to avoid such mistakes. While initially sceptical about VRE, he became a VRE advocate upon seeing himself 'do the wrong thing'.

What video makes visible and tangible then is that individual clinicians' actions are as likely to be an expression of their specialty's habits, team expectations and local care standards and facilities, as of personal intentions, decisions and abilities. Of course, in cases where clinicians suffer from excess fatigue, experience conflict, engage in unusual risk taking or display intense emotion in the face of suffering or an incident, you may capture things that are 'off the scale' in terms of general standards and accepted norms. However, you are more likely to encounter ordinary *problems*: patients not being discharged in a timely manner when services do not line up, personal protective equipment not being readily available when it is needed, or patients not being given the opportunity to contribute to handovers of care. Other problems you may capture include excessive noise in the workspace making it difficult to conduct medical or radiology rounds, frequent interruptions making it difficult for nurses to concentrate on preparing medications, problems with equipment delaying procedures or the risks of cross-contamination from the bags that doctors carry with them during their rounds.

The most common problem you will see is invariably to do in some way or another with troubled communication. It is noteworthy in this regard that non-communication and sub-standard communication among clinicians play a role in most reported incidents (US Joint Commission, 2011). Due to their ubiquity, you are likely to capture these problematic kinds of communication, as we did in our studies.

Other objections to your VRE study may include clinicians' and managers' preconceptions about scientific methodology. In health care, it is common to regard 'rigourous' (read: fixed, inflexible) scientific methods as guarantors of truth and others as inferior. The methods favoured tend to include first and foremost the randomized control trial and its various offshoots. You will need to have arguments ready, which will convince your audiences, that different methods are research-worthy because they yield different and new insights. Specifically, video footage provides a perspective on *in situ* practice that no trial can replicate. Naturally too, VRE's research questions will differ radically from the ones that underpin quantitative studies. Instead of pursuing context-free generalizable truths, VRE pursues context-specific learning and innovation. As noted, VRE harnesses complexity as a resource rather than trying to eliminate it as a problem.

Finally, the impact of video footage on people's awareness and agency will only become fully apparent to your audiences once they experience seeing themselves, or others, in situations and interactions with which they are deeply familiar. In anticipation of that, it is worth asking people if they have experienced viewing themselves on video engaged in a sport, playing with their children or even just walking, and then asking people what they remembered upon seeing themselves carrying out those activities. They may say, as many we approached did: those images have stayed with me, they have taught me a lot about my own and others' behaviour.

2.4 PROJECT DESIGN

Think about the design of your project as early as possible. As a participatory methodology, VRE projects will not be 'fixed' or fully mapped out from the start, even if you have created such a plan in order to apply for funding. In order to attract funding and have your study ethically approved, you will need to be able to articulate the study design and plan clearly and logically. In Chapter 1, we discussed the role(s) of the researcher and practitioner in VRE projects from a theoretical and methodological standpoint. In practice, you and your collaborators – whether they be clinical, research or public – will need to manage both the formal plans and detailed programmes you submit to funders, and the unpredictability that will inevitably characterize how your relationships and achievements with services, professionals, managers and patients will unfold.

To create structure for your project, you should ask the following questions. Who will lead and facilitate the work? Will it be you as a clinician, social scientist, health service researcher, quality improvement officer, clinician manager or research student? Will you invite (and perhaps train) clinicians to work alongside you, or will you take charge of the filming, checking the footage, editing the clips and organizing the reflexive meetings? What are the pros and cons of having medical clinicians, nursing clinicians, allied health clinicians or patients and families as collaborators? How do their respective profession-specific 'subcultural' stances (Degeling et al., 2003) bear on how to navigate around people's expectations and sensitivities? What are the pros and cons of having clinicians from the participating site running or contributing research time to the project? Will clinicians be released from their clinical work to be able to work on the project, or is their participation voluntary? Will you need to budget payment for their time into your grant application?

Further, if the project is to be driven and managed by clinicians themselves, do they have the governance structures, experience, equipment and resources needed to do so? Another important question is, how will you as a researcher or as a clinician ascertain whether your initiative has accomplished anything? How will you provide evidence of it having accomplished anything? What does measurement mean in the context of a flexible approach to improvement? What will happen beyond the project and how will it be sustained? These kinds of questions are critical for you to think about and develop answers to when preparing your funding application. Possible answers will appear throughout this chapter and throughout the rest of this book. The matter of evaluating VRE projects is addressed in Chapter 7.

One way of initiating VRE projects is the following. Our university teaching and talks at conferences put us in contact with clinicians and clinician managers who become interested in our ideas and thinking. They are happy to become our collaborators on grant submissions. We budget for one or two research nurses and a similar number of doctoral students. The project focus needs to be sufficiently critical for senior management to endorse the project (e.g. hospital-acquired infections, or handover and ward round communication), and to be of interest to two or three clinical sites, such that the project does not remain too narrowly focused on one ward or site only. The project outputs are framed in terms that appeal to clinicians, patients, service managers and policy makers (e.g. 'lowering hospital-acquired infection rates', 'raising handover and ward round information sharing efficacy and consistency'), and they may appeal to the interests of non-health funding agencies ('this study investigates what is collective competence and how it can be nurtured', 'this study demonstrates that video feedback strengthens professionals' agency and decision-making').

On the other hand, if you are a student wishing to use VRE in a masters or doctoral project, you may wish to draw on your (or your supervisors') connections to find one or more suitable sites, depending on your research question. Such projects run by one person alone would be more limited in scale and would have to persuade not only collaborators and participants of their value but also an academic audience, in relation to their value as pieces of research work. Finally, if you are a clinical nurse educator or a junior doctor who wants to use VRE to improve handover in a ward, for instance, then you already have your site and your topic, and your first tasks would be to persuade your colleagues, and to figure out how you might be able to resource your project in terms of equipment, and, most importantly, your time and your colleagues' time to participate.

Further, VRE studies can be tied in with other ways of gathering and analyzing data. The project's overall methodology may involve not just videoing and visual feedback but also thorough participant observation, an interview component, a survey component, a clinical outcomes measurement component allowing for statistical processing or a policy development component of interest to those in the domain of clinical governance and risk management. The project plan would set out timelines, milestones and delivery dates, in the knowledge that most projects (and not just video projects) have trouble meeting those exact commitments.

Finally, the project proposal may be enriched by a dose of adult learning theory, team/group dynamics theory and complexity theory, the main components of which were set out in Chapter 1 of this book, and which we will return to at times in what follows. Adult learning theory legitimates VRE and opens up its research potential through raising questions such as this: Does VRE strengthen team cohesion and collaboration, and can this be evidenced through demonstrating its impact on incident rates? Team dynamics theory may be invoked to ask questions about collective competence and distributed intelligence: Does VRE enhance inter professional communication and can this be demonstrated interactively and clinically? Complexity theory enables us to argue that conventional scientific approaches no longer suit the problems that professionals and patients encounter in health care. A new research paradigm is needed that acknowledges that complexity radically changes the improvement imperative. This new paradigm brings people together, less to gather knowledge about the past than to explore how to create new futures – might we call this 'pro-search' rather than 're-search'?

2.5 ATTRACTING RESEARCH FUNDING

We have attracted funding to carry out VRE projects from a diverse range of sources. In Australia, funding has been secured from both the national health and medical research funding body (the National Health and Medical Research Council) and the agency that funds social, economic and humanities projects (the Australian Research Council). Funding has also been obtained from a national health policy agency (the Australian Commission on Safety and Quality in Health Care) and from various state governments. In the Netherlands, health providers have themselves supported VRE in their hospital settings (Maastricht). In Utrecht, funding obtained from EU sources was used for a VRE project focusing on clinical handover. In the United States, video ethnography is undertaken and funded by Kaiser Permanente and more recently by the Mayo Clinic. In the United Kingdom, projects have received funding from the Economic and Social Research Council and the Wellcome Trust. Numerous doctoral projects are under way around the world with funding from a variety of sources: research studies, national government scholarships, as well as private funding. Examples of funded grants are included in Appendix A.

For the most part, a successful VRE grant application is no different from any other research grant application. That is, VRE grant applications will target the right funding body and show understanding of the priorities of that funding body and of the panels of experts reviewing the applications. The application will be tailored to the specific funding call and will be discerning about what the funder will or will not fund. The application will effectively address the research problem you have outlined; it will show the research is necessary, significant and feasible, and it will demonstrate there is a clear plan for the dissemination of findings, a solid project evaluation and a critical assessment of the sustainability of its outcomes. Finally, the research team is shown to have the skills and capacity to carry out the proposed project (Aldridge and Derrington, 2012). All these criteria speak for themselves.

As with the audiences you need to persuade to come on board with your project, funders may view VRE as unfamiliar and therefore as unproven, and they may therefore see all kinds of problems and challenges with what you are proposing to do. Project reviewers may not be familiar with or fully understand the philosophical justification for VRE (Iedema, Mesman, and Carroll, 2013). Their worldview may still be that a large sample size and the rigorously scientific and 'objective' discovery of generalizable knowledge should be the paramount aim of any funded research endeavour.

Funders may not appreciate that complexity demands new approaches and new pedagogies for acting more effectively and with greater impact in the contemporary world. They may underestimate how knowledge and evidence inevitably need to be contextualized, deliberated, adapted, modified, updated, refined, expanded and possibly overturned in the light of *in situ* experiences and locally emergent circumstances. They may still regard all this adapting, revising, deliberating and so forth as 'merely' a matter of 'translating' knowledge into practice, not realizing that the term 'translation' does not begin to capture the complexity of what is at issue here for front-line professionals and patients. All this puts you in the tricky position of having to speak the still dominant scientific (if not indeed 'positivist') language (language that posits a 'positive' and one-to-one relation between what it says and the reality it describes), while knowing that your project will unfold according to different principles and priorities.

Even if they accept that what you are proposing has value, funding agency expert panels may view your video-reflexive research as 'mere' local practice improvement, or as quality improvement, applying only to local service circumstances and local individuals without sufficient relevance for what people do elsewhere. Relying on what Dekker refers to as Newtonian thinking (Dekker, 2005), these panels may view knowledge dissemination still as a simple and linear process: we find out what works, we publicize our findings, we instruct local actors in what to do and we monitor the effect of this on their behaviours. Unfortunately, this line of thinking ignores local complexity and the need for local adaptability and flexibility.

Put differently, the complexity theoretical principle that the generation of knowledge and intelligence can no longer be constrained to being produced only in laboratories, and that it needs to be produced also where complexity is encountered, experienced and tackled, has not yet fully taken root. People may claim to have accepted complexity theoretical principles, without in fact realizing and internalizing the full array of implications of doing so. To overcome these obstacles, you need to maximize the significance, order and impact of your proposed initiative.

Aside from this, funders' attention may be piqued by how well you argue two kinds of justification. First, working with individual clinicians in a limited number of sites does not restrict your efforts to only affecting your participants' behaviour and their personal learning. Here you need to theorize the significance of perturbing local activity, thereby creating a dynamic that produces bottom-up innovations from insights and realizations that are more far-reaching than any single, local change. This impact goes beyond any particular improvements that result, as it includes the *learning* that has occurred, the different ways of seeing practice, and the strengthening of professionals' confidence and of their agency over how they work individually and in teams. In reference to the aphorism about *teaching* someone to fish as opposed to just giving them a fish, you leave healthcare professionals and patients not just with a fish (a new solution or improvement), but with a new approach to fishing (new approaches to producing improvements), and even with a way of multiplying the number of fish upstream (a general capacity for learning that will apply not just to your current focus [e.g. handover], but to anything that might warrant attention and improvement in the future).

Your second justification is that complexity means unpredictability and change. For this reason, complexity in health care increasingly demands that people *interact* and *communicate* with one another, as doing so will ensure they stay abreast of what is most current, effective and strategic, on the principle that 'more brains are better than one'. To develop this argument for your proposal, you need to frame healthcare safety or improvement as being not principally a technological or even technique-based endeavour, but principally a social, inter-personal and communication-based endeavour.

Communication may be scriptable and robots can now perform it, but ultimately the effectiveness of human communication is proportional to communicators' quality of conduct and their self-insight. Conduct and self-insight are reflexive dynamics performed in the moment – a far cry from communication produced from scripts or static algorithms, and from information issued by 'experts elsewhere' who have established communication scripts and interaction rules. (Even though artificial intelligence now enables machines to 'learn', machines are not very good yet at negotiating uncertainty, or at interpreting non-communication.) It is important to mention then that video-reflexivity calls professionals' and patients' attention to their local communication habits and assumptions, and that this enhances their practical intelligence by strengthening their insights into the *in situ* conduct of self and others. This learning process moreover is not simply a linear one, nor is it always measurable in terms of what people now know. Enhanced insight and awareness affect people and processes in complex ways that are not always predictable or knowable beforehand, nor are they easily measurable afterwards.

2.6 WHAT SHOULD BE INCLUDED IN THE PROJECT BUDGET?

Budgets for VRE projects may include salary calculations for research staff, and this can range from accounting for chief investigators' time commitments to the project to full- or part-time salaries for researchers, and possible stipends for doctoral students. Budgets should also include funds for equipment: video cameras, tripods, perhaps special lenses and long-distance microphones, laptops, speakers, video-editing software licences and portable storage drives or other storage solutions. A third important budget component concerns ethics applications, in case HRECs charge for processing your applications. Fourth, there may be travel costs, and perhaps accommodation and board costs, enabling research staff to access sites and spend time there. Lastly, budget items may include transcription costs, footage editing costs, administration support costs and research dissemination costs (open access publication payments to journals, conference registration costs, etc.).

2.7 RESEARCH ETHICS AND VRE

All research proposals are subject to ethics approval, and VRE can present particular challenges with regard to obtaining ethics approval. HRECs and IRBs may be concerned by the nature of the settings and the kinds of people you are proposing to involve in your project. Healthcare services are home to people classed as vulnerable: patients, most centrally, but also vulnerable populations amongst staff. Patients may not be deemed, by these ethical governing bodies, to be able to make competent decisions about whether to be involved in your research. Then there are the risks deemed to be associated with capturing healthcare workers' clinical activities. Some of these activities may refer to private matters or personal issues, and others may involve risk-taking and non-ideal or unfortunate outcomes that might not be deemed to be suitable for wider consumption and dissemination. All these things pose challenges that ethics committee members may not be inclined to ignore.

The ethical implication of this last sentence is worth exploring before we move on. At times, ethical concerns are deployed to deny access to organizations to conduct VRE. At other times, its scientific basis is questioned. Keep in mind that VRE is, in essence, a means to enable professionals and patients to scrutinize how care happens and bring how care happens more in line with people's expectations. Further, VRE is not about top-down performance or risk management, nor about catching people out, nor about incrimination, but about helping people broaden their engagement with and influence over what care is at any given moment. VRE is about learning, not blaming or judging. Framed thus, VRE may pose risks by revealing how care is actually done. These are not risks to patients so much as for clinicians and managers and services: what are highlighted are opportunities – obligations? – for improvement. As such, VRE is inherently an ethical endeavour, aiming to enhance people's ways of being and acting in the world.

If you are using VRE as a quality improvement tool in your service, for example, and use it as part of 'everyday' practice, responding to ethics committees' questions and concerns might be more straightforward, even when local ethics committee members are not familiar with VRE. Your project will clearly be governed by guidelines set by your healthcare setting. Conversely, you may be working with patients and families and follow them across multiple settings. This raises other challenges. To help you navigate these issues, we describe next the ethical approaches we have applied and include some of the frameworks which have helped to guide us in Appendix B. We also highlight resources and guidelines others have used in their approaches to using visual methods. Further, we outline some of the more common questions asked of us, both in the 'practice' of VRE and by Institutional Ethics Boards. Finally, we provide some examples of ethical dilemmas from our own experiences of using VRE and how we responded to them.

2.7.1 Institutional ethics versus 'ethics in practice'

The principles that inform regulatory approaches to research ethics in most Western countries are concerned with deontological and/or consequentialist forms of argument including minimizing harm, respecting the autonomy of participants and preserving their privacy and anonymity (Hammersley and

Traianou, 2014). Here, your study is held to be ethical if its outcomes are meliorative. In addition, and despite the significance and recognized importance of qualitative research in health care, many researchers feel their research is evaluated by review committees who are often more familiar and comfortable with quantitative designs underpinned by narrowly-defined scientific assumptions and favouring a rigourous (read: inflexible) methodology anchored in biomedical aspirations for knowledge and progress (Murphy and Dingwall, 2001; Boser, 2007).

In these conventional environments, clinician and patient participants tend to be regarded as potentially vulnerable subjects who need to be protected by 'a codified set of procedures that assumes a standardised, researcher-driven model of scholarship' (Martin, 2007: 321), rather than as individuals capable of engaging in a 'collaborative and negotiated research process' (Martin, 2007: 322) on their terms. It is noteworthy that in this view of participants as 'vulnerable' subjects, researchers become constructed as a 'threat' from which services, clinicians and patients may need to be protected.

Despite progress over recent years in healthcare research towards greater recognition of methodologies other than trials and conventional qualitative research, ethics committee members still tend to require you to describe methodologies in detail, plan your studies down to the month if not the week and outline any ethical issues you will encounter right up front. These expectations do not sit easily with how participative research tends to unfold. On top of this, innovative qualitative research frequently involves blurring boundaries that are deemed sacrosanct in the eyes of those adhering to more conventional views. This is not an argument in favour of vagueness. On the contrary, it is an argument in favour of ongoing communication, both with the ethics committees and with those providing consent.

For instance, ethics committee members may not be clear about the rationale underpinning researchers and research participants collaborating on data collection and data interpretation. In endeavours such as participative research, appreciative enquiry and VRE, research involves gathering not just accounts reconstructing what happened but also insights and interpretations ('analyses') from all involved to assist with devising new ways of going forward. Another boundary is blurred, therefore, by researchers and research participants when co-designing and redesigning the research as it unfolds, and this too can be uncomfortable for ethics committee members.

To rehearse the points made earlier in this book, our arguments supporting these boundary-blurring approaches, *in situ* adjustments and *ad hoc* decisions come down to this. Undeniably, the world (and therefore health care as well) is becoming increasingly complex. Complexity challenges what we know and how we habitually do things. Therefore, complexity should not be left to 'experts elsewhere' applying specialist techniques for illuminating complexity from a distance, and in doing so, providing elegant descriptions, neat generalizations and formal analyses that then require 'translation' into everyday reality. Rather, complexity must be tackled where (and when) it manifests itself in people's lives, such that people's ability to intervene in here-and-now complexity can be enhanced.

The principal research question therefore is not 'How can we understand and model complexity?', because answers to this question may be out of date by the time they are printed and out of sync with contemporary or local circumstances by the time they are applied. Instead, the principal research question is 'How can we all (researchers, research participants) become better at recognizing and negotiating complex situations?' This latter question can only be addressed by targeting and strengthening everyone's *in situ* responsiveness to complexity and their receptiveness to learning.

Another challenge may be seeking institutional ethics approval for multi-site qualitative research projects or participatory projects (Iedema et al., 2013). This can be a lengthy process taking up to 6 months or even longer, depending on your project design and on how many sites and jurisdictions are involved. Seeking approval from multiple ethics committees can result in different committees raising different, and at times contradictory, concerns in response to your project. For example, one committee may question your request to video patients, whereas another committee may question your decision *not* to video patients from culturally and linguistically diverse backgrounds. Both queries are valid, but they highlight that ethics committees may have divergent reactions to what you are proposing to do. It may appear though at times that committees are 'positioned in opposing moral universes that construe ethical research in very different ways' (Halse and Honey, 2007: 345).

Nevertheless, it is helpful to remember that both researchers and ethics committees have the same goal of ensuring that research is fully ethical. The specification of what 'ethics' means in the context of your proposed study may be difficult, but it is also invariably illuminating, as it asks you to articulate your assumptions, expectations and principles. We have always found this process rewarding in the end – particularly when approval was ultimately granted! We have successfully negotiated formal ethics processes for a diverse range of studies, which, at first sight, may have seemed too challenging from an ethical committee perspective. For instance, we have had studies approved where we involve vulnerable people, such as patients receiving palliative and end of life care (Collier and Wyer, 2016); people receiving critical care by ambulance staff, in emergency departments and in intensive care units (Carroll et al., 2008; Iedema et al., 2012; Hor et al., 2014); people with cognitive impairment; people in neonatal intensive care units (Mesman, 2015); people affected by HIV and AIDS (Thomas, 2011) and people from linguistically and culturally diverse backgrounds.

For its part, the notion of research and/or images as being harmful or distressing for participants tends to be based on the idea that participants are having the research done 'on' rather than 'with' them. But harm is culturally, situationally and contextually determined, rather than being simple and straightforward (Pink, 2007). Dying patients may request for their interview footage to be shown to all those training to be clinicians, as was true in our case (Collier, 2013). Others may be happy for footage to be shown to one group of people in a particular setting but not to another in an alternative setting. A staff member may be comfortable having a clip shown to their trusted team members in a reflexive session on their own ward, but may be less inclined for the same clip to be shown at an international conference, or vice versa. Others may be happy to allow anyone to see their footage. Participants' views often differ, and their views may evolve over time.

Thus, there is the ethics of negotiating your relationship and your uses of footage with participants, and there is the ethics of gaining formal ethics approval for your study. These dynamics may not fully align. This does not mean that you can tell participants one thing and ethics committees another. Rather, it means that you need to frame your ethics application in such a way that you have enough 'leeway' to allow you to revisit the bases of your agreements that you have struck with your participants. The overarching principle here is that you respond in general terms to ethics committee questions and concerns – general enough for you to retain a degree of freedom for how you structure your relationships and understandings with participants.

2.7.2 Negotiating VRE with ethics committees

Most generally, to obtain approval for your study, and where possible, try and cultivate a positive relationship with ethics review committees (Cartwright et al., 2013). This may involve you requesting an audience with your committee(s), to enable members to experience your passion for the aspect of care you are seeking to address, and hear your reasoning about wanting to deploy unconventional research. It is always helpful to get to know the committee chair and seek an interview with her/him, particularly when you do not have the opportunity to address the full committee face-to-face.

Also remember that the key to a successful VRE ethics application is to pre-empt what the ethics committee(s) will ask you and what might be of concern for them. The VRE community now has quite a stock of knowledge about ethics committee questions and concerns (go to the 'International Association of Video-Reflexive Ethnographers' website). For example, in a recent application to research in a unit caring for people with cognitive impairment, one of the authors drew on the work of Jan Dewing (2007) on 'process consent' (Dewing, 2007) to persuade the ethics committee that the research team's approach to gaining consent to video interactions between patients and staff was consistent with the committee's standards and expectations.

To help you navigate these issues, we have compiled a list of questions that ethics committees are likely to ask you and some possible responses (see Table 2.2).

2.8 ETHICAL FRAMEWORKS FOR VRE

Clark (2012: 25) argues that many of the ethical dilemmas that we are deemed to face as researchers using visual methods arise largely from 'a legacy of biomedical, or at least positivist-orientated, ethical principles that fail to fit with their predominantly post-positivist methodological frameworks'. VRE is post-positivist in orientation, insofar as it does not posit a one-to-one relationship between knowledge (or even data) and reality. We might qualify VRE even as a 'post-method' or a 'post-qualitative' methodology, due to its open-ended, under-determined

Table 2.2 Questions from ethics committees and possible responses

Questions to anticipate from your ethics committee(s)	Examples of responses you can give
To whom will you show the video footage?	Only those members of the research team listed in the ethics application will have access to raw footage. Otherwise, any identifiable footage shown during the research will depend on the permissions given by those who feature in the footage. Identifiable video footage will only be used for research dissemination if the participants who feature in the footage have consented for the footage to be shown externally, and have signed a media consent form, with the understanding that there are no consequences for declining to consent.
How will you make sure patients and family's confidentiality is maintained?	'Raw' footage will only be accessed by research staff. Approval will be sought from those featured before showing identifiable footage to other research participants. Footage used for wider dissemination will be de-identified, unless written consent for showing un-de-identified footage is obtained from those featured.
What if someone not associated with the project gets 'hold of' the footage? or what if footage ends up on YouTube?	VRE projects come with strict governance processes to oversee how footage is handled and stored in secure devices and locations, and who can access it.
What if someone is accidentally captured on film without their permission?	This may occur, and there are three ways of dealing with this. First, the activity and videoing are paused to alert the person to the videoing and to ask for their consent. Second, permission is sought post hoc from the person or people who is/are included in the footage. Third, if the above are not possible, the footage is erased.
Who will own the footage when you finish your project?	The university through which the project was conducted will be the owner of the original data, and the responsibility for safeguarding the footage lies with the project's Principal Chief Investigator.

(Continued)

Table 2.2 (*Continued*) Questions from ethics committees and possible responses

Questions to anticipate from your ethics committee(s)	Examples of responses you can give
Where will the footage be stored?	The footage will be stored on a password-protected computer or password-protected external hard drives, which are in turn stored in secure university (or hospital) offices. Footage may also be digitally stored in secure university research data stores.
Who will decide how the footage is used when the project is finished?	The responsibility for safeguarding the appropriate use of the footage lies with the project's Principal Chief Investigator. The Principal Chief Investigator will seek further permissions from those in the footage and from the institution's ethics committee if new uses for the footage are proposed that do not figure in the original ethics application, consent forms or 'media release' statements.
What will you do with footage that captures professionals doing the wrong thing, or doing things wrong?	Such footage will be retained, unless those involved withdraw their consent. Its use (or non-use) needs to be negotiated with the people in the footage. We obtained a footage of an ICU Director being involved in handing over information about the wrong patient. The Director requested a copy of the clip in question and showed it at several (international) conferences, stating every time that video reflexivity is critical to teams becoming alert to problems that they might otherwise dismiss as not particularly significant.
Will your footage be subpoenable?	Footage is per definition subpoenable. However, it needs to be emphasized that footage invariably reveals the complexity of *in situ* practice and, with that, the *social essence* of practice. That is, footage reveals what people do and say as being *prefigured* by how the institution works, and not just as issuing from them personally. Footage may therefore relieve individual actors of full responsibility for how activities unfold. In sum, footage in general, as well as footage of inappropriate practice, is more likely to alleviate than exacerbate individual people's personal responsibility for what goes on, as footage foregrounds the *social-institutional* and *cultural-historical* dimensions of what goes on.

approach to framing and conducting research. Framed thus, VRE's philosophy stands in stark contrast to the thinking that underpins conventional approaches to research that sweat replicability. VRE is in the first instance about engaging with people's lifeworlds without prioritizing disciplinary frameworks and procedural perspectives, and without predetermining the specific outcomes of such engagement (Iedema and Carroll, 2015). Only secondarily is VRE concerned about rendering its processes and impacts as formal knowledge.

Framed thus, VRE challenges ethics committees because of its open-endedness, and its reluctance to define up front what it will do and where it will go. In your ethics application, of course, you have to show that you have clear ideas about your approach and where you are hoping to go. This is even when you know that your VRE project will 'distribute agency more generously and less parsimoniously' (Law, 2004: 151) than might usually be the case, rendering your project subject to the mangle of participants' preferences, interests and concerns. Overall, VRE seeks to democratize the research process, and this may not sit well with those who privilege conventional ideas about researcher roles, research processes, objectivity and the role, purpose and meaning of knowledge.

Perhaps to counterbalance VRE's quite radical pursuit of research democratization and procedural openness, we have tended towards an ethically conservative framing of our work. This is the final and critical guiding principle of VRE: to *care* for our participants and to be attentive to their psychological safety (Edmondson, 1999) when we do VRE. For instance, we usually ask people's permission to show footage to specific audiences and for specific circumstances unless a person has made it clear that they allow the footage to be used anywhere and anytime by anyone. We err on the side of caution, and ask people twice rather than just once, and engage them in conversation to ensure they have a sense of what drives VRE, why we use video, how we understand 'analysis' and why we would ask permission for others to see the footage.

In addition, researchers need to be mindful of how to use culturally sensitive images. As a researcher working with the Australian Aboriginal community using visual research methods, Fran Edmonds stresses the importance of ensuring that appropriate members have granted permission for use of specific images. Some images, she notes, may be culturally sensitive if they include sacred material or images of the deceased (Cox et al., 2014: 14). Further, where a participant has died, unless that person has made it known that they wanted their clips to be shown, we should no longer show those clips. Where a person did originally give their permission, we have, in addition, consulted the patient's family members for consent *post hoc* for showing and using the clip.

This process of iterative and ongoing consent may need to be tailored to each participant in terms of when and how they wish to be consulted (Cox et al., 2014: 13). By the same token, having undertaken the study with their legacy in mind and having received their consent for footage to be shown to anyone and anywhere when they were alive, the researcher may then have to take it upon themself to show the relevant clips widely and to as broad an audience as possible.

The answers to questions about what to video and what not, whether to video an event or not and whether to show footage to particular people or not are never straightforward. We have struggled with these questions throughout all our projects. As VRE aims to democratize the research process, it regards the footage as being co-created, and, thanks to the primacy of the reflexive process, it regards the footage as also to some extent being co-analysed, depending on how the project unfolds. This approach is not equivalent with one where researchers collect information for specialized analytical purposes and which therefore is more like 'taking something away from participants' (Pink, 2007).

Inevitably though, images in which we appear take something away from us. This is particularly evident in situations where we become aware of images being used for purposes of which we were not informed. Some of us may have had photos used for conference brochures without being made aware of this in advance. In cases where video footage is used that portrays us, and where we have lost control over that footage, we become conscious of the risks associated with unfettered access to visual resources. As authors of a book on video reflexivity, we have agonized over what kinds of visuals and clips to include in the book and whether we have appropriate kinds of permission to include them. How might participants feel about an image being made public in several years' time? Might they regard the image as unrepresentative because they have moved on or changed in how they look? Might they accept our use of their images in cartoonized form?

The response that we can blur, pixelate or cartoonize images and footage to ensure confidentiality and preserve privacy is also not straightforward, however. While blurring footage may protect people's identity by removing 'their face', doing so may risk dehumanizing (or 'erasing') participants. If the blurring, pixelating or cartoonizing is not negotiated and agreed, doing so denies participants the opportunity to decide for themselves whether to reveal their identity (Cox et al., 2014). Although practically challenging, the best approach is for researchers and participants to keep in contact, and update their understandings and decisions about what is done and what may be done with the images and clips. This ongoing consent process is most likely to ensure 'informed consent', insofar as it keeps participants continually informed of the emerging ways in which their footage is edited and shown, and of the conditions of their participation.

On a broader front, our approach to ethics and ethical research practice is less about risk management, identity protection or adherence to rigid rules and regulations, than it is about an ongoing process of reflection, deliberation and agreement. In Appendix B, we describe some guiding frameworks on which you might draw for engaging in those negotiations. We have applied these frameworks to help us think through matters of ethics and ethical dilemmas as they have arisen in our numerous projects.

2.9 CONCLUSION

This chapter has described approaches to persuading services, professionals and patients to participate in VRE. We described tactics for designing proposals and obtaining project funding. We have also touched on the concerns held by ethics committees in the face of videoing care, and we have outlined optimal responses.

In our experience, it takes time for ethics committees to become comfortable with and understanding of VRE's approach, and we may need to enter into dialogue with them.

Overall, it appears that interest in how clinicians do their work in local settings is on the rise, in recognition that formal guidelines and policies are not reliable predictors of what happens in the name of care (Iedema et al., 2006). This rising interest in the actuality of care notwithstanding, commentators continue to promote methodologies that objectify and 'freeze' the processes of care for the sake of their elegant representation in reports and articles.

What these commentators lack is knowledge about and experience with approaches that make those processes come to life for those enacting them. These latter approaches highlight the complexity of these processes and credit front-line actors with being able to strengthen care practices 'from the bottom up'. As we have argued thus far, involvement of professionals and patients in scrutinizing care as it happens in this way is critical for producing meaningful, ethical and impactful changes in care, as well as practical and sustainable improvement outcomes across health care generally.

REFERENCES

Aldridge J and Derrington A. (2012) *The Research Funding Toolkit: How to Plan and Write Successful Grant Applications.* London: Sage.

Boser S. (2007) Power, ethics, and the IRB: Dissonance over human participant review of participatory research. *Qualitative Inquiry* 13: 1060–1074.

Carroll K, Iedema R and Kerridge R. (2008) Reshaping ICU ward round practices using video reflexive ethnography. *Qualitative Health Research* 18: 380–390.

Cartwright JC, Hickman SE, Nelson AC, et al. (2013) Investigators' successful strategies for working with institutional review boards. *Research in Nursing & Health* 36: 478–486.

Clark A. (2012) Visual ethics in a contemporary landscape. In: Pink S (ed) *Advances in Visual Methodology.* London: Sage, 17–36.

Collier A. (2013) Deleuzians of Patient Safety: A Video-Reflexive Ethnography of End-of-Life Care. PhD Thesis. Sydney: Faculty of Arts and Social Sciences. University of Technology.

Collier A and Wyer M. (2016) Researching reflexively with patients and families: Two studies using video-reflexive ethnography to collaborate with patients and families in patient safety research. *Qualitative Health Research* 26: 979–993.

Cox S, Drew S, Guillemin M, et al. (2014) *Guidelines for Ethical Visual Research Methods.* Melbourne: Visual Research Collaboratory, University of Melbourne.

Degeling P, Maxwell S, Kennedy J, et al. (2003) Medicine, management and modernisation: A 'danse macabre'? *British Medical Journal* 326: 649–652.

Dekker SWA. (2005) *Ten Questions about Human Error: A New View of Human Factors and System Safety.* Mahwah, NJ: Lawrence Erlbaum.

Dewing J. (2007) Participatory research: A method for process consent with persons who have dementia. *Dementia* 6: 11–25.

Edmondson A. (1999) Psychological safety and learning behavior in work teams. *Administrative Science Quarterly* 44(2): 350–383.

Halse C and Honey A. (2007) Rethinking ethics review as institutional discourse. *Qualitative Inquiry* 13: 336–352.

Hammersley M and Traianou A. (2014) An alternative ethics? Justice and care as guiding principles for Qualitative Research. *Sociological Research Online* 19(3): 1–24.

Hor S, Iedema R and Manias E. (2014) Creating spaces in intensive care for safe communication: A video-reflexive ethnographic study. *BMJ Quality & Safety* 23: 1007–1013.

Iedema R, Allen S, Britton K, et al. (2013) Out of the frying pan? Ethics approval for multi-site qualitative research projects. *Australian Health Review* 37: 137–139.

Iedema R, Ball C, Daly B, et al. (2012) Design and trial of a new ambulance-to-emergency department handover protocol: 'IMIST-AMBO'. *BMJ Quality & Safety* 21: 627–633.

Iedema R and Carroll K. (2015) Research as affect-sphere: Towards spherogenics. *Emotion Review* 7: 1–7.

Iedema R, Jorm CM, Braithwaite J, et al. (2006) A root cause analysis of clinical error: Confronting the disjunction between formal rules and situated clinical activity. *Social Science & Medicine* 63: 1201–1212.

Iedema R, Mesman J and Carroll K. (2013) *Visualising Health Care Practice Improvement: Innovation from Within*. London: Radcliffe.

Law J. (2004) *After Method: Mess in Social Science Research*. London: Routledge.

Martin DG. (2007) Bureaucratizing ethics: Institutional review boards and participatory ethics. *ACME: An International E-Journal for Critical Geographies* 6: 319–328.

Mesman J. (2015) Boundary spanning engagement on the neonatal ward: Reflections on a collaborative entanglement between clinicians and a researcher. In: Penders B, Vermeulen N and Parker J (eds) *Collaboration across Health Research and Medical Care*. Farnham: Ashgate, 171–194.

Murphy E and Dingwall R. (2001) The ethics of ethnography. In: Atkinson P, Coffey S, Delamont S, et al. (eds) *Handbook of Ethnography*. London: Sage, 339–351.

Pink S. (2007) *Doing Visual Ethnography: Images, Media and Representation in Research*. London: Sage.

Thomas V. (2011) Yumi Piksa: Community-responsive filmmaking as research practice in highlands Papua New Guinea. Unpublished PhD Thesis. Sydney: Centre for Health Communication, University of Technology Sydney.

US Joint Commission. (2011) The New Joint Commission Standards for Patient-Centered Communication. US Joint Commission.

3

Recruiting participants for video-reflexive ethnography initiatives

3.1 INTRODUCTION

There are many ways to do video-reflexive research once you're in 'the field'. In the following chapters, we present a broad overview of initial research activities, which broadly map on to what are usually seen as recruitment and data collection phases. Methodologically, video-reflexive ethnography (VRE) seeks to exnovate every-day practices *reflexively* and in *collaboration* with practitioners and stakeholders. Rather than prescribing a set of methods or procedures therefore, VRE accepts the need for flexibility in the face of *in situ* complexity. Thus, what drives your decision-making as the project unfolds will include: (i) the practical options and opportunities available in the research setting, (ii) your research questions and (iii) VRE's four general principles regarding exnovation, reflexivity, collaboration and care. This section delves more deeply into the basis of this advice, using our own experiences of conducting VRE projects in multiple sites and different ways.

To some extent, this chapter works off the assumption that you already have obtained formal approval to begin your research, including ethics, governance, site/security clearance and other relevant approvals, depending on your particular organizational context, and as discussed in Chapter 1. However, we acknowledge too that it is often the case that you may have to determine how you will perform the following activities in order to obtain those approvals.

Particular activities in which a video-reflexive ethnographer is likely to engage when in a field site include the following:

1. Recruitment (or, more accurately, explaining your project to those who you hope will participate)
2. Videoing practices (what we call data co-creation, as opposed to data collection)
3. 'Analysis' as an iterative, collaborative and interpretive process
4. Organizing and conducting reflexive sessions

This chapter and Chapter 4 concentrate on items 1–3. Chapters 5 and 6 will concentrate on item 4: the task of organizing and facilitating reflexive sessions with participants. Although we will discuss these issues in the above order, the recursive and iterative nature of some VRE projects means that sometimes recruitment, videoing of practices, analysis and reflexive sessions can happen concurrently or in any order rather than in a linear fashion. This is especially the case once the project is under way: new participants may be recruited continuously, early reflexive sessions may lead to different practices being videoed and analysis throughout may lead to changes in foci and in modes of participation.

Also, in some VRE projects, the video footage may be viewed immediately after the activity is recorded. More often though, there is a time lag between videoing practice and selecting clips. In each case, there are different considerations, such as the nature of consent given by those featured in the footage, choosing what to show, the practice aspects captured, effects of time, familiarity and who gets to see the footage. Our exposition may be sequential, but your project's unfolding may depend on how each of these issues works out in practice.

3.2 ENTERING THE FIELD: GAINING SUPPORT FROM AND RECRUITING PARTICIPANTS

At various points in your research, you will be called upon to explain your research to a variety of audiences in a persuasive manner in order to get their approval or gain their involvement. In Chapter 2, we explained how to deliver a 'sales pitch' to persuade senior staff and front-line professionals to sanction your research study and your presence in their organization. At this point, you have your project funded, and now you need to approach front-line staff, patients and/or patients' loved ones and invite them to participate. Largely, we have found that it is useful to develop a presentation that can be given in a variety of ways – ranging from a full 15–20-min presentation (maybe even with slides) to a captive audience of potential participants in a meeting room, to a quick and opportunistic 2-min chat with a key person you have just bumped into, and who has been difficult to pin down for a meeting. This is particularly important when your audience is unfamiliar with VRE and wary of the use of video.

In healthcare environments especially, there are often multiple research projects underway that ask staff to contribute their time and effort outside of their usual work, and this can lead to a sense of 'research fatigue' (Clark, 2008). Some staff may view new projects as 'yet another thing we have to do', so developing a well-designed presentation is important for informing and reassuring potential participants of the process and benefits of engaging in VRE. We suggest that the following kinds of information are included in your presentation, highlighting in particular the kinds of information that participants have most frequently asked of us.

3.2.1 Elements of a VRE presentation inviting people's participation

a. *Introduce yourself*: Who you are, where you are from and why you are here

It may sound obvious, but before you launch into talking about a project or the introduction of VRE into a healthcare setting, it can be helpful to explain who you are and your own interests in this study. For example, are you a clinician researcher? A social scientist? A student? Is this your PhD project? Are you a hospital quality improvement officer? Further, is this a government-funded project? By what organization or university are you employed? If you are initiating a VRE project in your own healthcare workplace, you will need to explain the background or context for your research idea and your motivation for choosing VRE.

It is also useful to inform potential participants of other stakeholders involved in the project, for example, other departments or disciplines who are part of the research team or who have sanctioned the study. You may also want to explain what ethics approvals have been obtained. Potential participants might feel reassured knowing that their managers and colleagues (if a staff member) or their healthcare providers (if a patient/family member) support the project; however, this can also bring up issues of power and the pressure to participate. These issues will be discussed further below.

b. *What is this study about*: What is the problem? What is the aim of the research?

This explains the need for the study, and depending on who your audience is, it should be explained in a way that is relevant to them personally and/or professionally. Generally, VRE projects are initiated from a widely recognized concern (e.g. clinical handover, infection control), but these concerns are put to potential collaborating practitioners and/or patients in the form of questions, to establish whether these foci are of concern to them. This may lead to discussions that highlight what are local concerns: how the night team hands over to the day team, or how the junior doctors hand over information compared to other doctors. In other words, the aims of the research and the problems targeted are explored with your audience rather than categorically stated.

c. *Why a different approach (VRE) is needed*

By describing the other approaches that have been undertaken to address the above problem, you can demonstrate a gap that VRE is designed to fill. Usually, VRE can be contrasted readily against methods that are too distanced (in time or space) from everyday practice to inform or change everyday local practice. Other methods may define the problem too narrowly and therefore underestimate the complexity of everyday healthcare practice. Or methods do not engage with the experience and expertise of front-line staff/patients, or only do so as part of initiatives that do not have ready access to decisions and discussions about how local care processes are organized, changed and improved.

d. *Explain VRE*: The principles, the methods, and what it looks like

To explain VRE, you can draw on the many arguments presented thus far and on ones that are yet to follow to guide your explanation. Box 3.1 provides an excerpt from an infection control project information sheet aimed at surgeons working in an acute inpatient surgical unit.

You can also include some examples of previous VRE projects. Depending on your audience, a copy of one or two relevant VRE articles can be helpful for illustrating VRE as a novel and well-established and creditable methodology. The Australian Commission on Safety and Quality in Health Care website also hosts a page with information and resources about a VRE project called Handover: Enabling Learning in Communication (for) Safety (HELiCS) (Iedema and Merrick, 2008; The Australian Commission on Safety and Quality in Health Care, 2018). The HELiCS VRE project was designed to enable front-line staff to monitor and enhance their own clinical handover practices and, in collaboration with more than 150 medical, nursing and allied health clinicians and patients, produced a professional video-reflexive resource that can be used in all manner of healthcare locations. Even if your project is not about handover, the HELiCS resources are full of visual images and example projects that are helpful for showcasing how VRE can be implemented. HELiCS includes a useful film portraying three services where improvements were achieved using VRE (www.youtube.com/watch?v=3EHOX6iAGUY).

Another useful strategy is to prepare a bank of short clips that can be shown at information sessions. This allows potential participants to better understand what the process of VRE will 'look' like. If you have never conducted VRE, there are examples you can access in some published papers (Iedema et al., 2015; Wyer et al., 2017). Alternatively, there are links on the *International Association of Video-Reflexive Ethnographers (VREIA)* website. If you are unable to show footage, it can be useful to use the analogy of elite athletes and sports people watching footage of themselves to better understand and improve their performance.

BOX 3.1: Segment of project information sheet that explains VRE to clinicians

VRE: A NEW APPROACH TO INFECTION CONTROL

VRE is a method that combines ethnography (the observation and analysis of practice) with the use of video as a learning tool. This method gives front-line staff the opportunity to reflect on their everyday practices, using video footage of those practices. Researchers work with participants to video their routine work, which may include ward rounds, insertion of devices and other procedures identified by participants. Selected clips are played back to staff in 'reflexive sessions' to allow them to view their own practices from a different perspective. Staff are invited to reflect on and discuss how they interact with each other, with patients and the environment, and to consider ways in which they can improve efficiency and safety.

This observation, feedback and reflection process represents a critical learning opportunity for clinicians. Seeing themselves on screen helps clinicians to appreciate dimensions of their work of which they may not have been aware. The visual experience, moreover, directly affects clinicians' sense of self and enables them to connect what they see directly with how they work *in situ*. At the same time, the visual data provides a rich picture of current ways of working, enabling clinicians to devise solutions to practical problems that they may not be able to conceive of while immersed in day-to-day practice. To date, VRE has produced improvements in clinical teamwork processes, clinical handover and infection control practice.

For this project, the focus is on infection prevention and control. The use of video is centred on learning, and is negotiated and carefully edited to avoid any focus on individual wrongdoing. Consent from participants is always obtained before videoing their practices or feeding back footage featuring them in reflexive sessions.

We will also invite patients and carers to be involved in the interviews and videoing, focusing on their experiences, informational needs and communication practices with healthcare workers. With their consent, video footage created with patients may be shown back to staff, to provide feedback about the needs of patients with multidrug-resistant organisms as well as the roles they may play in infection control and prevention.

e. *What's in it for them?*

While it can't always be known in advance what benefits participants will get from being involved in a project, you can talk to them about benefits participants in other projects have experienced. For example, healthcare staff who have participated in VRE projects have commented on how they appreciated being offered the opportunity and time to reflect on their own practices. Participants also appreciated being treated as experts of their own experiences and practices, and being offered the opportunity to share concerns and potential solutions with peers and managers. Patients and family members have also appreciated being given a space to voice their positive experiences, concerns or opinions about, and solutions to, healthcare quality and safety.

We have found that when clinician-researchers (Hay-Smith et al., 2016) are shown published, peer-reviewed articles on VRE projects, they can see the benefits of VRE not only for addressing local issues but also as a way to engage in research, which can add to their own professional metrics (i.e. to be research active). Similarly, we have also found that potential participants become more open to becoming involved in VRE projects when you discuss other high-profile organizations who have conducted VRE research (e.g. Mayo Clinic, Deaconess Health System and St Josephs-Exempla in the United States; Westmead Hospital, Royal Prince Alfred, Prince of Wales Hospital and Melbourne Health in Australia; and The Maastricht University Medical Centre and the University Medical Center Utrecht in the Netherlands).

f. How you are going to manage consents

As explained earlier, the learning opportunities offered through VRE require some vulnerability on the part of participants. It is therefore important that potential participants are assured of your commitment to providing a safe environment should they decide to participate. We suggest that you make the following clear to potential participants. The first two in particular are basic principles for all research involving human participants:

- Participation is voluntary.
- Participants can withdraw from the project at any stage.
- Even after formal written consent is obtained, verbal consent will be negotiated before any videoing occurs and participants can ask the camera to be turned off at any time.
- Verbal consent will also be obtained before any footage is shown back to other parties.
- You might also mention which human research ethics committees have provided formal ethics approval.

Formal ethics approvals and written consents may not be required, such as for internal quality improvement projects conducted within hospitals. This will depend on the policies at each healthcare organization. However, we suggest that a model of ongoing verbal consent, as described earlier, helps ease participants' discomfort with being videoed and ensures that they are able to consent to each step of the process. See Section 3.4 for further details regarding a model of 'ongoing consent'.

g. How long the project will last

Let participants know how long the project is likely to last, how often you will be present in their ward, department or facility and (roughly) when reflexive sessions will be offered. It can be useful to offer a timeline (see Figures 5.1 and 5.2 for examples), albeit emphasizing the collaborative nature of VRE projects, and that the project may unfold differently from how it was planned, acknowledging time, availability and funding limitations.

h. What kinds of outcomes and impacts you anticipate

You may be asked about the outcomes and impacts that your study may produce. Here you need to be clear about your intentions without committing yourself to achievements that are overly specific. What you can do at this point is point to the outcomes and impacts produced by similar studies (see Chapter 7 for a discussion of evaluation and research impact). Vignette 3.1 describes a study that aimed to understand what was successful interprofessional communication between a pathology unit and a surgical team. The study enabled each team to not only view the inner workings of their own practices, but for the first time truly grasp and positively appreciate the hectic and highly complex work of their colleagues in another department. This provided them with the opportunity to improve interprofessional communication by being able to collectively consider both sites of practice at once.

You may also like to use the example presented in Vignette 3.2. Patients and family members benefited from gaining a greater understanding of infection risks

---

**Vignette 3.1   A study to understand interprofessional
communication**

Title of project	Successful inter-team collaboration in surgery and pathology
Researchers, institution	Katherine Carroll (Australian National University, Canberra, Australia) and Jessica Mesman (Maastricht University, Maastricht, the Netherlands)
Funder	Mayo Clinic
Aims of study	To understand successful interprofessional communication practices between a pathology unit and a surgical team
Participants	Pathologists, pathology assistants, technicians (pathology) and surgeons, surgical assistants, surgical nurses (surgery)
Field site	Mayo Clinic, Minneapolis, Minnesota, USA
Description	In this project

- The surgical and pathology teams were invited to view and discuss video data of their own intra-team communication practices (separately).
- They were then invited to view and discuss video footage of inter-team communication practices (together).
- Participants were given the opportunity to identify what worked well for their own team, and what they appreciated about the other team's work in terms of how it assisted their own workflow.
- The surgery and pathology team then worked together using video data to optimize three key areas of their inter-team and interprofessional communication practices, including standardizing how to communicate surgical specimen orientations between surgery and pathology, and creating scripts for clearer report back of results between surgery and pathology.

Publication	Carroll et al. (2018).

---

and reduced incidence of health care-associated infections, and staff developed better understandings of how patients might become more involved in infection prevention and control.

3.2.2 Tailoring your presentation to different audiences

Now that you have an idea of what to include in your presentation, consider different ways this information can be disseminated to potential participants. Here you can think of a 10–30-min information session held at different times to accommodate shift work and rosters, a formal patient information and consent form, a one-page handout, or an informal chat. In busy healthcare settings,

---

Vignette 3.2   A study involving patients in infection prevention and control

Title of project	Integrating patients' experiences, understandings and enactments of infection prevention and control into clinicians' everyday care: A VRE exploratory intervention
Researchers, institution	Mary Wyer (PhD study; University of Tasmania, Darlinghurst, Australia)
	Supervisors: Rick Iedema, Suyin Hor, Clarissa Hughes, Debra Jackson
Funder	National Health and Medical Research Council of Australia (Grant/Award Number: 1009178)
Aims of study	To assist patients and clinicians to explore the ways in which patients could become more involved in hospital infection control
Participants	Patients and nurses
Field site	A 66-bed surgical unit in a metropolitan teaching hospital in Sydney, Australia
Study design	In this project:
	• Patients were invited to view footage of their own clinical interactions with clinicians and to comment on their understanding of infection risks and infection prevention practices.
	• Patients were involved in choosing which footage/aspects of care they would like to be fed back to the nurses. Video-reflexive sessions were then held with the nurses who cared for these patients.
	• Here, the original footage was presented alongside the footage of the patient commenting on the interaction.
	• Staff developed better understandings of how patients might become more involved in infection prevention and control.
Publications	(Wyer et al., 2015, 2017; Wyer, 2017)

---

with rotating rosters and shift work, it can be difficult to reach everyone in face-to-face information sessions or at formal meetings. A poster on a wall or a one-page handout that can be easily distributed can start to spread the word about the project. Consider including a photo of those who will be conducting the research on the poster/handout, as this helps potential participants to identify you.

If you are invited to present at a team meeting, you may only have 5 min to garner interest in your project. Similarly, formal patient information and consent forms, which must adhere to ethics committee standards, can be long and arduous to read. Therefore, a one-page overview handout can be useful for giving potential participants quick access to your main points. Finally, develop a couple of sentences that describe the project and the methodology that can be used to engage people when there are time constraints. For example, you may be videoing a team procedure, and someone unaware of the project joins the team who needs to be informed about the project quickly.

A presentation to patients and visitors may or may not be different to that given to healthcare staff. If you are working with a patient and public organization or group that is actively involved in designing and implementing a project with you, your presentation may be very similar to that provided to clinicians. But if approaching a patient or relative at the bedside, you will need to adapt your presentation to their appropriate level, taking into consideration their individual needs, severity of illness, level of education and cognitive function. Vulnerable populations are not well represented in healthcare research (NHMRC, 2006; Sarrami-Foroushani et al., 2014), and these vulnerable people may find themselves inappropriately excluded from projects. With some careful planning and manoeuvering, we may be able to involve them. Ethics committee instructions will often refer to the following groups as vulnerable: people highly dependent on medical care and possibly unable to give consent, children, pregnant women, people with cognitive impairment, indigenous people or people from culturally and linguistically diverse backgrounds. Several of these categories might also apply to healthcare staff, and you may have other categories to add to the list.

3.2.3 Using your presentation for recruitment

Now that you have your presentation in different formats, you can start to use these to explain the VRE project to your participants. You are likely to start by talking to the manager and/or education officer of the wards or units where you will be doing your research. You will be able to gauge who is able to assist you in arranging information sessions and meetings where you have access to staff. Perhaps one or more of the managers and other staff might come on board as co-researchers with you, and they may accompany you as you meet with potential participants, lending your work additional local credibility. Keep in mind however that this may be inappropriate in some instances, if staff feel unable to raise concerns or decline participation if their managers and supervisors are so closely involved.

You can also negotiate at this point when and how often participants may like you to be present in the workplace. We have found most sites are happy for us to come and go as we please. However, some managers may like to keep a closer eye on research proceedings and after-hours visits may need to be prearranged. It is a good idea in any case to let the manager or in-charge of whatever site you are attending know you are there each time you arrive on site. Not only is it polite, but they will be able to inform you of the current climate of the workplace and how available potential participants might be.

If you are planning to do some video-reflexive exploration in your own workplace, you will know best how to spread the word about your project. However, if you are a researcher who is coming to a site with which you are not familiar, you will need to find ways to contact potential participants. You may, for instance, arrange to speak at team or interdisciplinary meetings, or at in-services where you can reach a larger number of potential participants. If you plan to show video footage at these introductory meetings, make sure beforehand that you have the right connectors and adaptors to connect your equipment to projectors in the room, or movie files that are compatible with the available computer equipment, so that your presentation will run smoothly. Have one-page handouts available for people to take away, and if there is time, you can introduce the consent forms and ask for written consent at this time.

In hospitals, we have found that the period of time just before or after handover can also be a good time to give a brief explanation of your project to healthcare staff. Make sure the person in charge of that shift is aware you will be attending. We have also found that when you are observing or videoing at sites, people will ask what you are doing, and this presents an opportunity for a corridor conversation about the project. Alternatively, you can approach staff yourself, if they do not appear to be busy, to introduce yourself and ask if they would like to hear about the project.

Whether you are having a corridor conversation or giving a 5-, 10- or 30-min presentation, remember that people are busy, so keep to the schedule you have been allocated, keep it concise and allow time for questions.

Until recently, the main focus of VRE has been to do research with health-care workers for practice change. A small but growing number of researchers are now inviting patients and family members to become actively involved in VRE research. As VRE research with patients and family members expands, we will no doubt see a multitude of different ways that they become involved. Till now, the main ways that patients have been involved in VRE research has been in ward or outpatient-based projects (Collier et al., 2015, 2016; Wyer et al., 2015, 2017; Collier and Wyer, 2015; McLeod et al., 2016; McLeod, 2017).

How you might approach patients and visitors often depends on facility policy or ethics approval. Sometimes, ethics committees or site managers will require that you approach patients and visitors through their healthcare work-ers. Others will allow you to approach patients and visitors directly. In any case you should check with whoever is caring for patients because they will know if a patient is feeling unwell, about to undergo a test or procedure or if the patient is confused.

We have found, however, that sometimes staff will suggest patients whom they consider would be willing and informative participants, and we then find this is not the case at all. At other times, staff may suggest a patient who they think is not appropriate, and the patient turns out to be most interested in participat-ing and has a lot to talk about. Some patients feel more comfortable if they are approached directly by the researcher as they can refuse participation more eas-ily than if being asked by their healthcare provider. Conversely, we have also found that some patients are more trusting of you and the research if a healthcare provider introduces you. You will have to make the call as to which approach is more appropriate.

As suggested earlier, you will also need to consider the informational needs of patients and their family members. For example, in one of our studies, a patient newly diagnosed with an antibiotic-resistant infection was given a patient information sheet by an infection control professional. It was only discovered later that the patient could not read. If people do not speak the language in which information appears, you need to consider how you will engage with them. Through an interpreter service? With translated written material? Ethics committees can require comprehensive, and hence long, participant information and consent forms which can be quite daunting for some people. We have found it is helpful to take the time to go through and explain each section of the form according to patients' preferences.

3.3 COMMON CONCERNS AND HOW TO RESPOND

As mentioned earlier in the chapter, busy clinicians can sometimes view VRE projects as 'yet another thing they have to do', and being able to talk about the benefits of participation can be helpful. However, their concerns are more commonly related to their professional behaviour being recorded and shown to their colleagues. Managing these concerns often comes down to consent and confidentiality. Some people may be concerned that the footage from the VRE project might be used as part of their own performance assessment/performance review undertaken by their employer. You may need to ask managers to reassure their staff that this will not be the case and inform participants that the only people who will have access to footage are the researchers. Much more common is the general objection to seeing oneself on video, based on the assumption this will be embarrassing, and that it will expose mistakes and missteps.

Sometimes, teams are wary of being videoed, having had bad experiences in the past, and they may be reluctant or even refuse to let you video. For example, in one of our VRE studies, a researcher found that the nurses were reluctant to participate in VRE due to a previous incident on the ward where a colleague had taken footage in the workplace and uploaded it to YouTube without their permission. Paying particular attention to the VRE guiding principle of care, VRE researchers should take great care not to compromise participants' trust.

We have found that patients are often open to participating in VRE projects, on the understanding that it will improve care for them and other patients, and assuming that they feel well enough to participate. Some want to be assured that footage will not end up on YouTube, and once this worry has been allayed, they generally become very engaged. We believe this is a happy result of the relationships of trust we actively seek to build with patients: taking time to explain the research, showing them the footage immediately after videoing, making decisions with them about what footage might be shown to staff and keeping them informed and updated about the research progress. Healthcare workers also bring up concerns about obtaining patients' consents, and they can be reassured with an explanation of how you will approach patients for their written or verbal consents. We have found that emphasizing the iterative consent process as set out in Section 3.4 can help to allay fears.

3.4 ESTABLISHING ONGOING CONSENT PROCESSES

Expanding on our discussion of iterative consent in Chapter 2 (Section 2.7), we should explain that we practise VRE drawing on the notion of 'situated ethics' (Clark, 2012), and this manifests in the form of a continuous consent process (O'Reilly et al., 2011). By this, we mean that consent given by a participant to be involved in VRE projects does not end with signing a formal written consent form, but is, by necessity, a matter of constant engagement at every stage of the process (O'Reilly et al., 2011). This is largely because, when participants agree to engage in research methods that they have not experienced before, informed consent cannot really be achieved at the outset. Participants cannot really know beforehand what it means to be videoed and to watch themselves back on screen with colleagues. Some may feel completely at ease about the process until the first time they watch themselves back on screen. Others may initially refuse to participate, not liking the idea of being videoed, or because they may be deterred by the formality of the language required by ethics committees in participant consent forms.

We find that some people come to feel more comfortable about participating after seeing their colleagues being videoed and/or after attending a reflexive session. As such, with VRE projects, it is necessary to treat consent as an ongoing process. Remember to continue asking participants for consent, throughout the project, and especially at crucial points, such as when you wish to use their footage for a reflexive session.

Sometimes, situations arise where videoing needs to begin before those featured have given formal written consent. An example of this was during one project, when a researcher was in the process of recruiting a patient who had verbally agreed to be videoed during a particular procedure. When the team performing the procedure arrived suddenly however, there was no time to obtain the patient's written consent. Instead, the researcher asked again for verbal consent to video the procedure and then obtained the written consent afterwards. You need to check whether this is an acceptable procedure for your ethics committee(s).

As noted in Section 3.2.1 on developing a VRE presentation, participants also need to be reassured about the safety of participating by being made aware that a one-off formal written consent does not provide a blanket consent to being videoed at any time and for any audience. Make it clear at the time of formal written consent that you will also seek verbal consent whenever their video footage is to be used. The following list is by no means exhaustive, but may give you an idea of when it might be appropriate to check again with participants for their consent for you to engage in the following activities:

- To observe/follow an individual/team
- To video their activities
- To keep the video
- To show the video to important others (e.g. managers)
- To show the video to colleagues during reflexive sessions
- To show the video to other members of the research team

In Chapter 8, we will address two further issues for which iterative consent may be required. These include consent for

- Showing the video (de-identified or not) at conferences.
- Using the video or clips (de-identified or not) in journal articles or books.

Regarding these last two points, a general media release form, separate to the research-specific participant consent form, can be useful for obtaining permission to use stills or footage at conferences or in publications. Many healthcare facilities have media consent forms that can be used for this purpose, and if not, you can create your own with the legal team at your facility. It is a good idea, however, to check with your relevant human research ethics guidelines for any local privacy restrictions on identifiable data.

Finally and most importantly, the more preparation time you allow at the beginning of your project for setting up relationships and allowing feelings of trust and respect to develop with participants, the more spontaneous you will be able to be about negotiating consent in the field.

3.5 CONCLUSION

This chapter has described strategies for recruiting participants, and it has outlined the kinds of argument you can mobilize to persuade people to participate. We suggested that you need to be prepared to tailor your presentations to different audiences: physicians, nurses, allied healthcare professionals, managers, patients, carers and a mix of all these. Each type of audience requires subtly different angles. Some expect formal evidence, 'sound' scientific studies or confirmation from authorities in the field. Others expect proof that video-reflexivity is more than people looking at themselves, and that it achieves real outcomes for patients and teams. Again others may want to hear about validity and generalizability. You need to be prepared to vary your angle depending on who walks into the room.

Chapter 4 moves on to the practice of videoing care practices. It addresses the technological, practical and relational issues that arise there. With this, we move from our office into the field: the service, the ward, the unit, the community centre, the polyclinic and so on. If our office affords us thinking and planning time, the field presents itself as a jumble of problems and challenges, tasks and questions. We will have to key in to the dynamics of service relationships and look for opportunities and sympathies. Up to now, we have had time to design and rationalize our approach at some distance from the reality of everyday care. We are now going to have to mobilize knowledge, arguments and insights while 'on our feet'.

REFERENCES

Carroll K, Mesman J, McLeod H, et al. (2018) Seeing what works: Identifying and enhancing successful interprofessional teamwork between pathology and surgery. *Journal of Interprofessional Care.* doi: 10.1080/13561820.2018.1536041.

Clark A. (2012) Visual ethics in a contemporary landscape. In: Pink S (ed) *Advances in Visual Methodology*. London: Sage, 17–36.

Clark T. (2008) 'We're over-researched here!' Exploring accounts of research fatigue within qualitative research engagements. *Sociology* 42: 953–970.

Collier A, Phillips J and Iedema R. (2015) The meaning of home at the end of life: A video-reflexive ethnography study. *Palliative Medicine* 29: 695–702.

Collier A, Sorensen R and Iedema R. (2016) Patients' and families' perspectives of patient safety at the end of life: A video-reflexive ethnography study. *International Journal for Quality in Health Care* 28: 66–73.

Collier A and Wyer M. (2015) Researching reflexively with patients and families: Two studies using video-reflexive ethnography to collaborate with patients and families in patient safety research. *Qualitative Health Research* 26: 979–993.

Hay-Smith EJC, Brown M, Anderson L, et al. (2016) Once a clinician, always a clinician: A systematic review to develop a typology of clinician-researcher dual-role experiences in health research with patient-participants. *BMC Medical Research Methodology* 16: 95.

Iedema R, Hor S, Wyer M, et al. (2015) An innovative approach to strengthening health professionals' infection control and limiting hospital acquired infection: Video-reflexive ethnography. *BMJ Innovation*. doi:10.1136/bmjinnov-2014-000032.

Iedema R and Merrick E. (2008) *HELiCS: Handover – Enabling Learning in Communication (for) Safety: A Handover Communication Improvement Resource*. Sydney: Australian Commission on Safety and Quality in Health Care & Centre for Health Communication – University of Technology.

McLeod H. (2017) Respect and shared decision making in the clinical encounter: A video-reflexive ethnography. PhD Thesis. University of Minnesota.

McLeod H, Bywaters D, Collier A, et al. (2016) The patient revolution and video-reflexive ethnography. In: *ACSPRI Social Science Methodology Conference*. University of Sydney, 19–22 July.

NHMRC. (2006) *Guide to Effective Participation of Consumers and Communities in Developing and Disseminating Health Information*, Canberra: Australian Government.

O'Reilly M, Parker N and Hutchby I. (2011) Ongoing processes of managing consent: The empirical ethics of using video-recording in clinical practice and research. *Clinical Ethics* 6: 179–185.

Sarrami-Foroushani P, Travaglia J, Debono D, et al. (2014) Implementing strategies in consumer and community engagement in health care: Results of a large-scale, scoping meta-review. *BMC Health Services Research* 14: 402.

The Australian Commission on Safety and Quality in Health Care. (2018) *HELiCS as a Tool for Ongoing Observation, Improvement and Evaluation of Clinical Handover*. Available at: https://www.safetyandquality.gov.au/our-work/clinical-communications/clinical-handover/national-clinical-handover-initiative-pilot-program/helics-as-a-tool-for-ongoing-observation-improvement-and-evaluation-of-clinical-handover/

Wyer M. (2017) *Integrating Patients' Experiences, Understandings and Enactments of Infection Prevention and Control into Clinicians' Everyday Care: A Video-Reflexive Ethnographic Exploratory Intervention.* PhD Thesis. Hobart: University of Tasmania.

Wyer M, Iedema R, Hor S, et al. (2017) Patient involvement can affect clinicians' perspectives and practices of infection prevention and control: A 'post-qualitative' study using video-reflexive ethnography. *International Journal of Qualitative Research Methods* 16: 1–10.

Wyer M, Jackson D, Iedema R, et al. (2015) Involving patients in understanding hospital infection control using visual methods. *Journal of Clinical Nursing* 24: 1718–1729.

4

Videoing and analyzing practices

4.1 OVERVIEW

This chapter sets out the process of videoing healthcare practices. We first describe the kinds of technologies you'll need. Following that, we discuss the different styles of videoing that are available to us. We then address the practical dimensions of storing video footage. The chapter concludes with a note on video-reflexive ethnography's (VRE) approach to analyzing video footage.

4.2 VIDEO TECHNOLOGIES

There is an increasing variety of video recording devices available to consumers nowadays. Unless you are planning to create a professional quality movie, you may be considering something more along the lines of a handheld consumer camcorder or tablet, a worn camera (e.g. lapel or head-mounted), or video camera-enabled glasses, and these are only some of the many possibilities commercially available. Most likely, you will be recording in a digital format and showing footage directly from your device or after editing your footage on a computer screen or via a projector onto a larger screen. With this increasing variety of videoing and display options comes a growing understanding of the implications of each decision. As always, costs, availability, acceptability to participants, and other practical constraints will determine your options (see Box 4.1 for some practical tips on choosing a camera).

As discussed in Chapter 1, the video camera is far from a neutral instrument producing a faithful version of the real (Bell and Davison, 2013). Inevitably, the camera will impose restrictions on vision in terms of angle, distance, width and so forth. That said, and as Lomax and Casey (1998) point out, the camera's non-neutrality is not a methodological flaw to be eradicated or even mitigated. This is because the idea that reality can ever be comprehensively captured on video is false. No amount of videoing can replicate the real. Instead, the camera's non-neutrality does require researchers' reflexive attention to how the video camera affects the activity being videoed and how it visually constructs that activity. For instance, do you video people in close-up (perhaps because there is limited

---

BOX 4.1: Issues to consider when choosing a camera

- Camera size – how visible can the camera be (or how unobtrusive does the camera need to be)
- Camera weight – weight can affect your own health and safety; holding cameras for long periods and across many days can put strain on hands, wrists, necks and backs
- Playback screen – you can review footage immediately on a reasonably sized display screen
- Battery life – spare batteries or power adapter should be available
- Quality of footage – professional quality footage requires a higher level camera
- Functionality – the camera can be carried/worn for 'point of view' shots or mounted on a tripod (or placed on surfaces)
- Sound – how necessary is capturing good sound for your project; how good is the built-in microphone, and do you need an external or distance microphone

---

room)? Do you use a low angle lens (looking up, because people are tall) or a high angle lens (looking down, because people are shorter than you)? Do you use a wide-angle lens (to widen your vision and capture more information) or an ordinary lens (because that is all that was available)?

Other relevant questions to think about when considering how videoing practice constructs 'the real' can be exemplified as follows: When might you start videoing a nurse performing a dressing change on a patient? Is it once the trolley and equipment are all collected and the nurse has washed her hands and is ready to touch the patient? Or does it begin with the nurse hunting down an available trolley, cleaning it and collecting dressing equipment from the store room? Or should you start even further back, when she checks in on the patient to see what dressing they currently have on, to determine what items she needs? At which points do researchers and participants consider the work of doing a dressing change to begin and end? Do hand washing and trolley cleaning count as part of the work, or is infection control to be categorically/conceptually separated from the dressing procedure?

Being reflexive about how choices such as these are made means attending to what is made present as well as what is excluded from (later) viewing. Keep in mind though that video footage is likely to be seen as 'hologrammatic' as we described in Chapter 1. That is, when viewed by those familiar with the videoed context, video footage enables them to bring into the picture and discussion that which is *not* shown: previous activities and events, concurrent activities and events, the future of what is happening, local norms and expectations, interpersonal relationships, the consequences of all these practices and events for quality and safety, and the opportunities for change. Thus, what is shown and what is not shown are not mutually exclusive. That said, what is shown may motivate viewers to extrapolate about some things, but not others.

Keep in mind though that it is realistically impossible for everything everywhere to be made visible. This is not a drawback unique to VRE but a fact that applies to all research (see Iedema et al. (2013: 178) for a response to the charge that this limitation may detract from VRE). The consideration that video will never capture everything everywhere does underscore the importance of being reflexive about how the videoing process is negotiated with participants. Anticipating our discussion in Section 4.4, we note that this reflexivity refers not only to *what* is videoed but also to the *styles* of videoing. For instance, the camera may remain in a fixed location, providing a 'fly-on-the-wall' panoramic view of a surgical theatre (Carroll, 2009; Mengis et al., 2017), a patient's room or an empty corridor in an ICU, where both nurses and patients are isolated behind closed doors in single rooms (see Figure 4.1). The camera may remain in a fixed location, set up on a tripod but closer, to record the interactions between a clinician and their patients (see Figure 4.2).

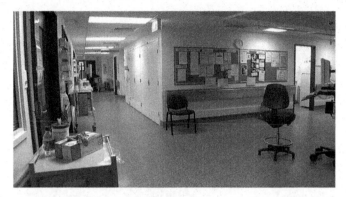

Figure 4.1 Fixed location camera. (Image courtesy of Su-Yin Hor, University of Technology, Sydney.)

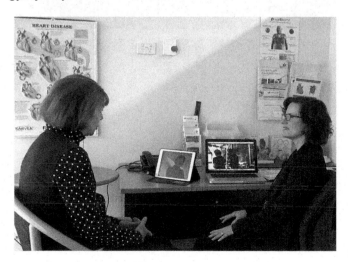

Figure 4.2 Camera placed on a tripod. (Image courtesy of Danielle Bywaters, University of Tasmania, Hobart, Australia.)

In her project about respect and shared decision-making in clinical encounters between patients and clinicians, McLeod used two cameras: one recording the patient and the other recording the clinician (McLeod, 2017). This generated different emphases, which she then used differently depending on the audience in the reflexive sessions that followed (see Figure 4.3).

The camera may also be handheld (or worn) by the researcher or participant (see Figure 4.4). This enables you to re-position yourself to capture the interactions between participants (e.g. a nurse executing a procedure in the incubator while colleagues comfort the patient, or a registrar being assisted by a nurse educator to set up a sterile trolley for central line insertion). A handheld or worn camera also enables you to track people's movements through space (such as a patient in their bed being pushed through the ward, or doctors conducting their rounds across wards).

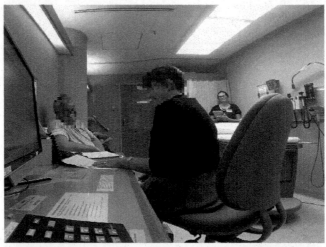

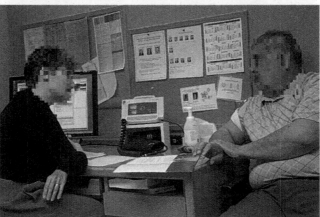

Figure 4.3 Two cameras, two perspectives, one event. (Images courtesy of Heidi McLeod, Geisinger Health System, Danville, PA.)

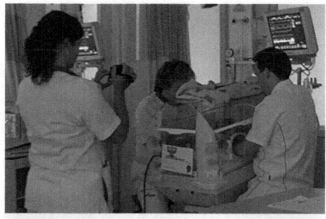

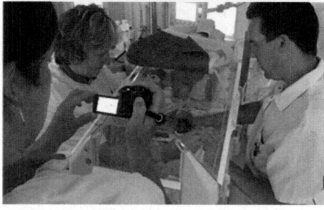

Figure 4.4 Handheld camera following actors and actions. (Images courtesy of Jessica Mesman, Maastricht University, Netherlands.)

4.3 UNDERSTANDING THE FIELD

If you are unfamiliar with a site, it is often helpful to start with a period of eth-nographic field observation and interviews. This can help you to understand who is who, how the site or field functions and what kinds of activities take place. It will also help you plan how to approach potential participants. For example, it helps you understand when the generally busy times are that might mean staff are unavailable, when patient rest periods are, when there are quiet times that can be conducive for interviews or for 'spontaneous' and *ad hoc* reflexive sessions and so forth. Interviews form part of the data creation and are helpful in under-standing the field site but can also assist in developing relationships of trust with participants that can lead to opportunities for videoing.

How long should you wait before asking whether you can video care practices? This will depend on how comfortable people are with being videoed but can also be influenced by the timeframe for the research project. Sometimes, we find that

---

BOX 4.2: Videoing emergency department handovers 24/7

Katherine Carroll, Jessica Mesman and Eamon Merrick were the researchers on a project that sought to capture emergency department handover practices 24/7. They initially attempted to do this on alternate 8-h shifts. After 2 days of trying this, they acknowledged it was impossible to juggle all the tasks they were required to complete: introducing themselves to all the patients and staff members involved in the handover, describing the project, gaining consent and then videoing. Sacrificing the aim of capturing footage during all hours of the day for the sake of capturing at least some footage well, they decided to change their approach. One researcher identified potential handover occurrences in the triage area and videoed the initial handover of the patient there. The other researcher set up inside the emergency department and gained consent from the doctor and nurse who were going to receive the patient. The first researcher was then able to video a smooth transition from the triage into the main emergency department (Carroll and Mesman, 2011).

---

staff, having heard about a project in an information session, are so engaged with the idea of video-reflexivity or the project aims that they ask you to video as soon as the project starts. Or it may be through the interview process that you find out what is important to a person or a team, and then you can suggest and negotiate a plan for videoing.

Some projects do not afford the luxury of spending a lot of time on observing and understanding the field. For example, Katherine Carroll and Jessica Mesman (2011) describe the challenges they faced working in a highly time-bound video project that sought to intervene in emergency department handover practices. As experienced hospital ethnographers, their usual practice of taking sustained periods of time to build trusting relationships with participants and to negotiate consent for videoing was challenged by a compressed and intense four-day period in which they needed to inform and consent participants as well as video handover practices. See Box 4.2 for how they managed this using a team-based approach.

It can also be difficult at sites with high patient turnover to find the time and opportunities to form relationships with patients and/or family members before asking them to be involved in videoing. Some researchers have addressed this by spending extended time, *after* videoing and reflexive sessions, building relationships with participants (Wyer, 2017).

4.4 STYLES OF VIDEOING

In a recent article, Mengis and colleagues demonstrate in depth how the different analytical lenses afforded by different video-recording 'apparatuses' (a combination of camera angle and movement) actively serve to configure the scenes and events videoed (Mengis et al., 2017). They demonstrate how different ways of using the camera serve to undermine the illusion we may have about video footage 'transparently' showing what 'happened'.

Likewise, LeBaron and colleagues describe the ways in which our 'cinematic decisions' – whether you turn the camera off at any time during recording, whether you use multiple cameras, whether you come into view of the camera and so on – may correlate with our assumptions and preconceptions about the practices and people videoed (LeBaron et al., 2017). The arguments put in these articles are relevant here, because they underscore our point that our cinematic decisions will highlight some features of the scenes and events we video at the expense of others. And this, in turn, is likely to have implications for how our footage is viewed, how it is responded to and how it is interpreted in reflexive sessions.

It is therefore important to be reflexive about the style of videoing you adopt and its potential consequences for the dynamics of your reflexive sessions. It may also be useful to experiment with different cinematic decisions, to alter the ways in which footage is collected and to consciously vary your cinematic decisions. For instance, besides videoing a team of doctors doing their handover by following near them, could you also video the handover from a patient's point of view, by standing next to the patient rather than next to the doctors?

You could also allow participants to provide a running commentary on their practices and environments to you holding a camera or into a participant-held camera. This is what Carroll (2009) refers to as 'expert-apprentice' videoing. Further interesting effects may come about if you invite the participants to turn the camera on you, the researcher. This happens, for example, when they want to demonstrate events like 'teaching a novice (the researcher) how to wear a protective gown' or to show (on the researcher) the contamination risk of dangling lanyards and identification cards worn around the neck. These examples demonstrate how boundaries can be blurred between researchers and participants as co-creators in the research. When participants are more active in directing the footage, they may experience a shifting of power relations, as is typical when deploying participatory methods (Gallagher, 2008).

Having said that, handing the camera to participants is not necessarily *better*. Participants may not wish to hold or direct or speak to the camera. Doing so may also not be feasible for them for practical (e.g. infection control) reasons. In fact, you should always take care with the camera and who holds it as it may turn into a cross-infection risk. While handing the reins (i.e. the camera) to your participants may yield interesting results, and while capturing their views and knowledge is important, you should not forego your own perspective on how clinicians and patients ordinarily enact their care. Our reason for saying this forms the crux of VRE: people's own views and professional-practical knowledge will rarely net in all the habits and customs that make up care as it ordinarily happens. VRE makes these habits and customs visible, and it does so precisely to strengthen people's ability to become aware of and intervene in the things they have 'learned to forget'.

As noted above, the 'hologrammatic' character of video footage refers to its potential to reveal for participants that which is *beyond* the video footage. They may be reminded of past actions which led to the visualized scenario, the sociopolitical relations and norms that guided the events, their own assumptions and habits and the possible or actual futures that (might have) eventuated from those scenes. We emphasize this hologrammatic aspect of video footage here to remind ourselves that what is shown forms only a limited aspect of what people will 'see'. In our experience, even small segments of footage enable participants to extrapolate into pasts, presents and futures. As said, we do not need to worry about being comprehensive since we will never capture everything.

Likewise, we dismiss the idea that video footage represents what really happened, referred to as the 'myth of transparency' (Bell and Davison, 2013: 175). The styles we choose and the cinematic decisions we make may inspire participants to engage with, and perhaps even intervene in, the taken-as-given dimensions of care. Our yardstick remains calibrated around engagement, deliberation and questioning, not proof and comprehensiveness.

In Table 4.1, we discuss how VRE guiding principles can assist you – in combination with your research interests, participants' interests and the practical constraints of your fieldwork – to decide how, when, where and what to video.

In Box 4.3, we present some practical advice for how to carry out videoing in a way that is comfortable for your participants and yourself.

Table 4.1 Guiding principles in deciding what to video

Theoretical principles	What/how to video
1. Exnovation	What: Routine and taken-for-granted activities How: Planned and opportunistic videoing
2. Collaboration	What: Practices identified by participants (e.g. as important, interesting, good or problematic) How: Invite participants to identify what to video, invite participants to do the videoing
3. Reflexivity	What: Aspects of practice that remain unquestioned How: Footage portraying practices from different points of view (e.g. from the patient's point of view); different examples of the 'same' activity
4. Care	What: Practices that participants are comfortable being videoed doing How: Consent as a situational, continuous process, requiring the researcher to be open and accountable to participants from the start and throughout, to be prepared to apologize where appropriate, to be contextually aware while videoing, to be spot, respect and respond to participants' discomfort

BOX 4.3: Practical tips for comfortable videoing

VIDEOING FOR YOUR COMFORT AND THAT OF THE PARTICIPANTS

- Locate a secure place to store equipment at the research site, such as a locker or a lockable room. Carrying a variety of valuable, heavy equipment (camera, laptop, audio recorders, etc.) on a person all day is not practical, but it is also not advisable to leave these in a public place (e.g. when you need to go to the toilet!).
- Source a good shoulder bag with pockets to store equipment you do need to carry around when looking for opportunistic moments to video (e.g. camera, pens, handouts, consent forms).
- Hold the camera away from your face (e.g. below or to the right or left of your face), so participants see your reassuring countenance (where appropriate) rather than the impersonal camera lens. This also allows you to maintain eye contact and communicate with others as a co-participant in the event, and lets you be aware of not just what the camera is recording but also the context in which the recording is taking place – so you might know, for instance, to stop recording if participants begin to look uncomfortable.
- Interact with participants while videoing to put them at ease – to suggest it's not so serious and to demonstrate that it doesn't have to be 'perfect'.
- 'Mute' sound recording if necessary by inserting an unattached jack into the microphone socket.
- Ask participants to direct the camera and guide the videoing.
- Consider beginning by videoing something less threatening, for example, asking participants to draw a map of their ward, and then videoing that drawing and their commentary.
- Always give participants the opportunity to see and/or delete the footage as soon as possible after videoing.

4.5 ADDITIONAL CONSIDERATIONS

You need to consider what you will wear during fieldwork. While you do not want to hide yourself or what you are doing, you also don't want to draw attention to yourself in such a way that people are distracted or confused by your position in the workplace. In the project described in Box 4.2, the researchers were asked by the clinicians to wear scrubs to help them blend in to the research setting. Similarly, if you are working in a setting where staff wears rather casual clothing, such as in some mental health units, wearing a suit might not be appropriate.

If you are entering patient care areas, you should make sure that you abide by infection prevention and control standards. Ties, scarves, lanyards and bags can become contaminated with disease-causing pathogens that can then be spread to other locations. Clothes that leave your arms 'bare below the elbows' allow you to wash your hands and wrists effectively between visits to different patients. If you are working with patients who are on particular transmission-based precautions, such as for multidrug-resistant organisms like methicillin-resistant *Staphylococcus aureus* or vancomycin-resistant *enterococci*, you will need to consider how you take research equipment like consent forms, audio-recorders, video cameras and laptops in and out of rooms.

Mary Wyer's research on patient experiences of infection prevention and control meant that she spent a lot of time in isolation rooms with patients under transmission-based precautions. She devised a system in which all equipment could be transported on a trolley. Before she touched anything on the trolley, she could wash her hands and the trolley itself could be cleaned before entering and after exiting the room. Similarly, in some places (e.g. operating theatres, neonatal intensive care units) where procedures are done, there may be certain areas that are considered sterile and which you may not be able to enter or use to put down equipment like cameras and notebooks. Speak with the managers of your field sites to discuss appropriate infection control behaviours.

Finally, another consideration, especially for clinically trained researchers who may be particularly observant, is to discuss ahead of time with managers what to do if you happen to observe something that concerns you. In healthcare settings, this may include serious (or potentially serious) patient safety breaches (Iedema and Piper, 2011). There may also be other instances when you observe or experience something that makes you feel uncomfortable or unsafe for any reason. As we mentioned in Chapter 1, VRE can be an uncomfortable and challenging process for researchers, and we suggest that researchers have support systems in place, whether with other members of the research team, supervisors or external parties such as counsellors, to help in debriefing and making sense of any difficult experiences during fieldwork.

4.6 MANAGING YOUR VIDEO FOOTAGE

Now that you have some video footage, this section discusses what you might do with it. It covers organizing and storing your footage, and establishing whether you have 'enough' video footage. Decisions about these matters will of course inevitably depend on your participants, the field site, your research interests, equipment and personal preferences. In what follows, we provide some general principles.

4.6.1 Storing and organizing footage

The best advice we can give is to organize your footage from the start – for instance, by date, location, participant and type of content (e.g. interview, footage of practices, footage of reflexive session, etc.) You may need to do this for raw footage, using your video editing software, as well as for the clips you create from that footage. Furthermore, it is good practice to download the footage as soon as possible onto *secure* storage (whether it be computers, external hard drives, servers or cloud storage), so that you can erase the footage from less secure cameras and free their memory up for new footage.

Keeping and regularly updating a fieldwork diary can help you to keep track of your activities and data created. Maintaining a fieldwork diary also assists in giving you a quick overview of what you have done, in terms of keeping track of dates, counting the number of interviews, adding up the hours of observation and so on.

When you have begun creating clips, and wish to get consent from featured participants to use them for reflexive sessions, it is helpful to have a secure device on hand (a laptop, tablet or phone) that you can use to show the clips at any time. Some participants may be comfortable with reviewing the raw footage immediately after being videoed, in which case a display screen on the video camera will be helpful. In either case, maintaining contact with participants is crucial, whether by collecting their contact details beforehand or by maintaining a constant presence in the field site.

4.6.2 How will I know if I have enough video?

Rather like a hologram, every small insight, question, or action leads to different ways of relating, which work from within, to influence the whole.

(Cunliffe, 2002: 40)

The answer to the question 'what is enough?' is rarely self-evident. Nevertheless, there are questions, based on VRE's four guiding principles, which can guide a self-assessment about how much footage you might need and whether you are ready to hold a reflexive session (see Table 4.2). You'll see that, in contrast to being governed by the conventional ethnographic principle of saturation (Morse, 1995), sufficiency of footage is determined by asking rather different questions: Not, 'does the research team deem sufficient visual data to have been collected', but, 'does the footage collected allow the four principles of VRE (exnovation, collaboration, reflexivity, care) to be realized'? (Table 4.2)

Your research interests will also provide a preliminary answer to your question about whether you have sufficient footage. Keeping in mind that participants will always see more than you show them, if you want participants to examine their practices for improvement, you may want to show them footage of them doing something that is unexpected, unusual, exceptionally interesting, or not as successful as it should be. When deciding what footage to use, we do not restrict ourselves to only that which is good or only that which is not. Besides, most if not all video clips will have some positive and some less positive facets embedded in them. You may further find that 'good' does not mean the same thing to everyone. Also remember that what looks like a problem to you may not look like something problematic to your participants, and vice versa.

Ultimately, our decisions about what to video and what to pursue should occur not just on the basis of technical concerns or formal plans but also on the basis of being mindful of our relationships, of the dynamics of those relationships and of

Table 4.2 Determining whether you have enough footage

Guiding principles	Questions to guide you in your assessment of whether you have sufficient video footage
1. Exnovation	Have I captured a range of activities/spaces in my video footage (or a range of different people doing similar activities/in the same space)? Have I got some footage of practices that showcase successful practices? Have I checked with practitioners and/or patients whether my footage captures interesting and representative aspects of practice?
2. Collaboration	Have I created opportunities for practitioners and/or patients to guide the videoing? Do I have clips of the activities in which participants expressed particular interest?
3. Reflexivity	Do I have clips that show different perspectives on an activity or practice? Do I have any clips that contrast (whether in content, point of view or variety) with what participants have been telling me?
4. Care	Are participants happy and consenting to me to keep videoing? How much videoing did I agree to do, and did I adhere to this agreement? How many clips do I have permission to show? Am I able to organize for videoed participants to be present at reflexive sessions, if they wish? Am I going to be showing footage of anyone who might feel more than usually vulnerable, in an audience of their colleagues?

the mood of the project and people's feelings about how it is going. It is generally helpful if you can ask one of your participants to help you determine if you have sufficient clips of interest to their colleagues. They may pick something up that you missed, and suggest you collect more footage of particular aspects of practice, or discard footage because what you have fails to reveal what it is intended to reveal. Still, be prepared for the possibility that their colleagues (those who turn up on the day) see things differently again. It may also be that what *they* are interested in is not what you've shown them, but different facets of practice that are only tangentially related to what you've shown them. The dynamics of these kinds of responses are discussed in Chapter 6.

In all, you have to be prepared to not be certain, ahead of time, about what people are going to say, and into what direction they may want to steer the discussion, or even your entire project. You can prepare extensively, but a clip that you (and perhaps others) find terribly interesting may elicit no more than a 'yup, that's how it is around here' on the day itself. A clip that you think is at best a bit of filler may, by itself, set off an hour of impassioned debate. Generally, however, due to the polysemic character of video footage, different people are likely to respond differently to the same clip. Their discussion is valuable: they may for the first time ever have the opportunity to hear colleagues' views on the technical, processual, social and emotional dimensions of their work.

Practically, it may be that you have to schedule the first reflexive session well in advance of knowing if you have enough footage. In this case, it can be helpful to fall back on the 'structure' provided by the principles above, especially if you have not had an easy time collecting footage. By focusing especially on collecting a range of clips of everyday ordinary activities, you ease the pressure on participants (and yourself) to either demonstrate or record something 'special' in your footage. One of the grounding principles of VRE is to refocus attention on the mundane as something that is special in its own right. Especially for a first reflexive session, this can assist participants in 'acclimatizing' to the sensations of watching themselves on screen, with their colleagues, and it allows the facilitator to gently scaffold the group discussion to elicit the nuances, complexity and accomplishment of their ordinary everyday activities.

Finally, the ethical dimension of choosing clips is perhaps the most important one. Apart from ensuring that you have the consent of the featured participants to show the clips, it is also important to consider if any participants are especially vulnerable in the setting. Patients and family members, for instance, are particularly vulnerable if they are currently (or will, in the future, be) dependent on the staff for treatment and care. Junior members of staff and casual or agency staff may also feel vulnerable having their behaviours scrutinized by colleagues, as may ancillary staff such as cleaners and porters.

Likewise, there may also be tensions between different teams or professions in the field site, and people may be critical of one another's practices. In these cases, the time you spend in the field site doing ethnographic observation and talking to people will help you to estimate if the intended audience will be supportive or unnecessarily critical when viewing the footage. If you are unsure, it may be better to err on the side of caution, and not show a clip that you feel presents a risk, or, preferably, schedule particular reflexive sessions (e.g. for specific groups only) so as to show the clips in a supportive environment in the first instance. Here, maintaining 'psychological safety' (Edmondson, 1999, 2004) for participants is crucial to making it possible for them to learn using VRE.

4.7 EDITING CLIPS FOR REFLEXIVE SESSIONS

As we move on to considering the editing of footage to produce clips to be shown at reflexive sessions, it may be worth reiterating that every stage of decision-making in the VRE process is an opportunity for what may be termed 'analysis'. For this book, we define analysis quite loosely. What we have in mind is along the lines of what Tavory and Timmermans describe as 'abduction' (Tavory and Timmermans, 2014). In essence, abduction provides licence for making creative connections among more or less similar phenomena. It is based on a 'form of reasoning through which we perceive the phenomenon (to be) related to other observations' (Timmermans and Tavory, 2012: 171).

This abductive process of creative reasoning gives you considerable freedom when choosing how to video practices as well as deciding how to edit your footage. It is useful to keep notes of any such abductions that occur to you as you conduct your study.

Returning to the issue of editing your footage, the principal questions that you will need to decide on are what to include and exclude, and how much. Should you show the entire sequence of an activity, or should you focus on only 'the main action' and cut out the 'dull bits'? The answer to such questions depends on what counts as 'the action' and to whom. Your reflexive session audience may find it stimulating to watch the entire length of time it takes to perform the activity in question, and they may well find the 'dull bits' fascinating.

As discussed earlier, the editing decisions you make will depend on your aims, the guiding principles and the practical considerations of the time you have available for reflexive sessions and the intended audience. For instance, if you are anticipating a large and diverse group in your reflexive session (more than ten people), and perhaps only 30 min for a session, then you may wish to prepare shorter 'activity-dense' clips of 2–5 min each, leaving more time for people to have their say. You can accomplish the same effect with a longer clip, but pausing every few minutes for discussion. If you have footage of a long (but relatively silent) activity, such as a nurse changing a dressing or a doctor performing a central line insertion, you can prepare longer clips and invite discussion as the clip plays.

Generally, however, it is better to make sure you have enough time for discussion during the reflexive sessions and to edit your clips for length accordingly. One particularly useful technique, especially if you wish the reflexive group to speak while the clip is playing, is to put in subtitles where you would like the audience to hear clearly what was said. We have generally, without special training (other than by going through YouTube tutorials), been able to use the readily available editing software that is associated with Mac operating systems, such as iMovie and Final Cut Pro. And there is an increasing variety of video editing software available to choose from. See Box 4.4 for some of the basic editing functions that we have found useful in preparing clips for reflexive sessions.

Finally, as required as part of your ethical approval, everyone who has been captured in footage that is being edited for a reflexive session needs to have given

---

BOX 4.4: Useful basic editing techniques for preparing clips

- Selecting, cutting and deleting sections of footage
- Inserting transitions between cut sections of footage: fades, black pauses, etc.
- Inserting titles and subtitles
- Blurring of faces (including moving faces)
- Exporting files to a variety of formats

their consent, but sometimes people will have walked past in the background, or the camera will have accidentally captured those who were previously out of view. In those cases, where the footage does not feature them but where you do not have their written consent or any means of contacting them, you may want to blur their features so that they are unrecognizable to your reflexive session audience. This blurring does not tend to work as well when it comes to footage of people's colleagues, as we have found that people are very good at recognizing colleagues from details as small as their posture or the type of shoe they are wearing. For those, it may be better to use only footage for which you have permission to show, rather than trust that blurring will be sufficient. A more comprehensive form of de-identification is to 'cartoonise' your footage. Premier Pro software allows you to apply all kinds of effects that render individuals and settings unrecognizable, including 'solarize', 'posterize', and 'colour emboss' (for an example, go to the Video-Reflexive Ethnography International Association website).

4.8 MAINTAINING PSYCHOLOGICAL SAFETY

The most critical thing to keep in mind when videoing people's practices is that you need to create and maintain a safe environment for all participants. This point can be framed by referring to Edmondson's (1999) conception of 'psychological safety'. Psychological safety happens when people feel able to speak up, without fear of being embarrassed, rejected or punished. In VRE, this applies as well to participants feeling safe about having their practices videoed and shown to colleagues during reflexive sessions. During the reflexive sessions, discussed in Chapters 5 and 6, participants then need to be able to admit to feeling their work warrants questioning, or needs improvement, for whatever reason. For VRE to proceed, participants need to feel able to discuss collectively and safely what they do, how they do it, and how it may be done differently.

Psychological safety is clearly critical for all those involved in healthcare research and improvement. Indeed, insofar as VRE is concerned, psychological safety is VRE's principal condition of possibility. If participants do not feel safe when enacting care and being videoed, or when discussing their conducts and activities as shown in the footage, it is unlikely that their subsequent discussions will engender the kind of reflexivity in the sense intended here. Critical to remember here is that psychological safety is not achieved once and for all; it needs to be nurtured and attended to constantly, with care, and without fail.

VRE researchers need to be on the lookout for dynamics or tensions that unsettle or threaten participants' safety. They need to attend to the risk that particular kinds of videoing or footage, or comments on footage, may make participants feel unsafe. They need to realize that psychological safety can never be assumed. Psychological safety may flourish as the project unfolds, or it may evaporate in response to single unsettling statements, reactions, events and developments. Without question then, psychological safety is central to VRE, and as concept it underscores the significance of relationships and interpersonal dynamics that are the heart of VRE (Iedema and Carroll, 2015).

4.9 RESEARCHER REFLEXIVITY

Another critical aspect of what is discussed here is the need for *researcher reflexivity* as the project unfolds. Researcher reflexivity is critical to VRE, since VRE does not regard the relationships between researchers and participants as arbitrary to research outcomes or to these findings' ability to 'travel'. VRE researchers' legitimacy can no longer be deduced from their role as researchers as such. Put differently, the way you position yourself as researcher will be proportionate to the outcomes you achieve. For example, a distanced, formalized and rigid stance may encourage a similar stance on the part of those who participate in your study, and it may therefore limit the degree to which participants are open to you and to your thoughts, perspective and findings. In contrast, a considerate and sensitive or *affective* stance may be more likely to engender interest in your work, your comments and your interests. Such a stance will be more inductive of participants accompanying you on your VRE journey.

In this context, the three-layered framework described by Nicholls (2009) provides a helpful way of thinking about VRE reflexivity, and in particular, researcher reflexivity (Collier and Wyer, 2015). While participants' reflexivity is the principal aim of VRE, researcher reflexivity is to be regarded as its 'mode of transport' if you like. Hence, and firstly, researchers are asked to consider the opportunities as well as the limits and opportunities that they themselves bring to the VRE collaboration. This involves researchers reflecting on their own positioning in all aspects of the research. This is *self*-reflexivity.

At the next level is interpersonal or *relational* reflexivity. This mode of reflexivity calls on researchers to evaluate their interpersonal encounters and capacities for developing relationships with participants. While VRE may be defined as a visual approach, it should be clear that its absolute point of gravity is human relationships and relationship dynamics. Conducting such relationships well depends on our capacity for relational reflexivity.

Finally, there is *collective* reflexivity. Collective reflexivity asks researchers to consider how the research process and design affect progress and findings, structure change outcomes and enable learning. Ultimately, the issue comes down to this: is VRE able to inspire in participants (and in researchers themselves!) a growing receptiveness towards complexity (Biesta, 2015)? As noted in our introduction, this last question is the crux of VRE. VRE is not principally about producing formalized knowledge, nor even about designing practical solutions, but about supporting people's growth and learning (including our own) to enable them (and us) to act with greater confidence and appropriateness amidst complex circumstances.

4.10 CONCLUSION

This chapter has set out the technological and procedural aspects of videoing *in situ* care. The chapter has also addressed how to manage footage and what questions to ask about the data you have collected. The chapter has further touched on what analysis means in the context of VRE. Finally, it has considered the critical importance of maintaining the psychological safety of participants and of practising researcher reflexivity in the interest of ensuring that relationship dynamics are such as to be able to mediate interests and insights. In Chapter 5, we move on to describing how to prepare for reflexive feedback sessions.

REFERENCES

Bell E and Davison J. (2013) Visual management studies: Empirical and theo-retical approaches. *International Journal of Management Reviews* 15: 167–184.

Biesta G. (2015) Freeing teaching from learning: Opening up existential pos-sibilities in educational relationships. *Studies in Philosophy and Education* 34: 229–243.

Carroll K. (2009) Outsider, insider, alongsider: Examining reflexivity in hospital-based video research. *International Journal of Multiple Research Approaches* 3: 246–263.

Carroll K and Mesman J. (2011) Ethnographic context meets ethnographic biography: A challenge for the mores of doing fieldwork. *International Journal of Multiple Research Approaches* 5: 155–168.

Collier A and Wyer M. (2015) Researching reflexively with patients and fami-lies: Two studies using video-reflexive ethnography to collaborate with patients and families in patient safety research. *Qualitative Health Research* 26: 979–993.

Cunliffe AL. (2002) Reflexive dialogical practice in management learning. *Management Learning* 33: 35–61.

Edmondson A. (1999) Psychological safety and learning behavior in work teams. *Administrative Science Quarterly* 44: 350–383.

Edmondson A. (2004) Learning from failure in health care: Frequent opportu-nities, pervasive barriers. *Quality and Safety in Health Care* 13: ii3–ii9.

Gallagher M. (2008) 'Power is not an evil': Rethinking power in participatory methods. *Children's Geographies* 6: 137–150.

Iedema R and Carroll K. (2015) Research as affect-sphere: Towards spherogen-ics. *Emotion Review* 7: 1–7.

Iedema R, Mesman J, and Carroll K. (2013) *Visualising Health Care Practice Improvement: Innovation from Within.* London: Radcliffe.

Iedema R and Piper D. (2011) The implications of mandatory notification for clinician-researchers involved in observational research in health services (letter). *Medical Journal of Australia* 195: 54.

LeBaron C, Jarzabkowski P, Pratt MG, et al. (2017) An introduction to video methods in organizational research. *Organizational Research Methods.* doi:10.1177/1094428117745649.

Lomax H and Casey N. (1998) Recording social life: Reflexivity and video meth-odology. *Sociological Research Online* 3: 1–26.

McLeod H. (2017) Respect and shared decision making in the clinical encoun-ter: A video-reflexive ethnography. PhD Thesis. University of Minnesota.

Mengis J, Nicolini D and Gorli M. (2017) The video production of space: How different recording practices matter. *Organizational Research Methods*. doi:10.1177/1094428116669819.

Morse J. (1995) The significance of saturation (editorial). *Qualitative Health Research* 5: 147–149.

Nicholls R. (2009) Research and indigenous participation: Critical reflexive methods. *International Journal of Social Research Methodology* 12: 117–126.

Tavory I and Timmermans S. (2014) *Abductive Analysis: Theorising Qualitative Research*. Chicago, IL: Chicago University Press.

Timmermans S and Tavory I. (2012) Theory construction in qualitative research: From grounded theory to abductive analysis. *Sociological Theory* 30: 167–186.

Wyer M. (2017) *Integrating Patients' Experiences, Understandings and Enactments of Infection Prevention and Control into Clinicians' Everyday Care: A Video-Reflexive Ethnographic Exploratory Intervention*. PhD Thesis. Hobart: University of Tasmania.

5

Preparing reflexive sessions

5.1 INTRODUCTION: WHAT IS A REFLEXIVE SESSION?

In our introductory textbook *Visualising Health Care Improvement*, we define video reflexivity as 'the practice of filming professionals at work and sharing with them the resulting footage with the aim of engendering discussion about their work' (Iedema et al., 2013: xviii). Reflexivity occurs when practitioners negotiate and gain new perspectives on their actions and decisions. A reflexive session is a meeting that aims to stimulate reflexivity. Such a meeting brings together the researcher, healthcare professionals, patients and/or others, and aims to elicit conversation about existing practices and relationships, spurred on by footage of actual behaviours and interactions.

Reflexivity here is not the same as reflection. We regard reflection as a personal activity that focuses the individual on their past. Reflexivity, by contrast, is a shared deliberation about existing circumstances and practices such that these are apprehended in new ways, thereby creating the possibility for new insights, new identities and new social and organizational futures (Iedema, 2011).

As video-reflexive ethnography (VRE) has evolved over the years, we have learned about what it means to have certain kinds of participants involved in reflexive meetings and what the likely dynamics of the meetings will be. That said, meetings are often surprising and unique. Our years of conducting VRE studies have enabled us to reflect on these dynamics, the kinds of responses people make to seeing themselves, the types of grouping, spaces and issues that encourage and those that tend to dampen discussion. This chapter and Chapter 6 describe our experiences and summarize our advice for optimizing the outcomes from the reflexive process. These two chapters will also provide examples of some of the ways that video-reflexive sessions have been conducted to date.

This chapter details how VRE's guiding principles – exnovation, collaboration, reflexivity and care – can inform the planning and conducting of video-reflexive sessions. Chapter 6 turns to the more practical aspects of organizing and facilitating reflexive meetings.

5.2 DRAWING ON GUIDING PRINCIPLES TO FACILITATE REFLEXIVE SESSIONS

Let us use VRE's guiding principles again to think through the various dimensions of running reflexive sessions. Before we do so, we should acknowledge that reflexive sessions can be challenging and unpredictable, but that they can also produce 'fireworks': staff experiencing realizations that hit them like lightning bolts upon viewing themselves and colleagues on screen. A frequent response is, 'Looking at this footage I realize how complex our work really is, and we do this every day and we just take it for granted'. Responses may also be more personal, such as those of an anaesthetist when watching footage of himself entering a busy operating theatre: 'Did I really just walk in there with a cup of coffee in my hand?!'[1]

5.2.1 Exnovation: Foregrounding the accomplishment and complexity of everyday practices

At the heart of the video-reflexive session is the process of exnovation. By creating a space for participants to view and comment on footage of their work, VRE enables them to 'exnovate': to become aware of and engage with the complexity of their everyday practice (Iedema et al., 2013). In our 2013 book, we defined exnovation along two dimensions. One is practitioners becoming aware of the actual *in situ* complexity of everyday work processes through viewing themselves on screen. The other is researchers eliciting ideas and insights from practitioners, and practitioners eliciting ideas from one another, about how to strengthen and enhance existing care practices, capitalizing on the things of which they are now newly aware.

Why is exnovation so central? Well, in our Introduction, we referred to front-line care as 'the zone of maximum complexity'. Care is the focal point for medical, nursing, allied health and managerial specializations; for guidelines, policies and protocols; for technological changes and resource constraints; for religious, ethical, practical, moral and political differences and for individuals' ambitions, fears, suffering and desire. And yet, when we ask people about what goes on during care, their responses are rarely comprehensive in how they portray and represent that care. This is not surprising, since most of human behaviour is anchored in habits, and habits tend to drop off our radar. In the literature, habits are described as behaviours that frame and structure the recurrent dynamics linking actors, purposes, resources and environments (Nilsen et al., 2012; Bennett et al., 2013; Grosz, 2013). Authors have different views on habits' potential for adaptation, but they tend to agree that habits become taken for granted and more or less 'automatized' over time, particularly if they don't encounter challenges or obstacles.

---

[1] We thank Liesbeth van Rensen and Bas de Vries for relaying this statement to us, Utrecht Medical Centre.

Undoubtedly, automatized habits are important for 'oiling' how we move through life. They relieve us of the burden of paying too much attention to habituated domains of life. If habits become fully automatized, we enact them unthinkingly. This means habits calcify and lose their adaptability, or their 'intelligence'. This happens because we stop monitoring their efficacy, and we choose to ignore the practical tensions they incur (Dewey, 1922). At this point, a gap opens up between what we do and what we choose to be conscious of. This is what motivates Greatbatch and colleagues to point out that 'there is often a gap between what people say and what they do' (Greatbatch et al., 2001: 189).

People are often unable to describe in detail even the most mundane of practices that they use and rely upon. In normal circumstances, these practices are tacit, taken-for-granted, seen-but-unnoticed, and are rarely discussed or even thought about (Greatbatch et al., 2001: 189).

Increasingly, the rapid pace of change in the contemporary world means that there is greater pressure on us to monitor, intervene in and adjust our habits. In the past, we have operated on the principle that adjustments to habits will happen gradually and automatically, as and when they are practically needed. But 'in today's increasingly complex and quickly changing world, environments are altered ... at rates far too rapid for effective unreflective readjustment of habit' (Shusterman, 2008: 211). Indeed, the modern world now demands that we reflect on and change ourselves *proactively* (Sloterdijk, 2013).

Aligned with that agenda, VRE pursues a reflexive re-adjustment of habit. VRE enables practitioners to raise automatized behaviours to awareness and therefore render those behaviours more malleable than they might otherwise be. To facilitate this process, VRE researchers choose video clips to show back to participants that will help them explore routine, frequent and often taken-for-granted, practices. This process of 'mild and moderated confrontation' with existing *in situ* practices captures the essence of exnovation. Through this process, we aim to uncover, with participants, their existing, everyday habituations and competencies. We do this with the view that participants scrutinizing their own practices in this way increase their agency and control over what is done, and working out whether things can or should be done differently (Iedema et al., 2006; Mesman, 2011).

That said, exnovation may be confronting for those who are disinclined to view themselves and their behaviour 'from under a different aspect' (Wittgenstein, 1953; Iedema et al., 2009b). People's identities may be invested in how they are and act in the world to such a degree that they are reluctant to change and unwilling to change themselves. This means that you have to take care with what you show back to people, as they may not always be receptive. We address the delicate dynamics of these exchanges in greater detail in Chapter 6.

5.2.2 Reflexivity meetings and collaboration

It is primarily during the reflexive sessions that participants' contribution is both most demanding and most exciting. These sessions offer participants the opportunity to come to terms with how much of their day-to-day behaviour is likely to be habitual. Indeed, this is the time and place where exnovation may be achieved: new viewpoints may emerge, and new realizations and new insights may occur. Keep in mind that there are many ways in which you can approach the collaborative design of your reflexive sessions, and that this will be influenced by your relationships with your participants and by what you hope to achieve through the session.

It may be useful to think about VRE collaboration as allowing for different modes. One is captured by the term *clinalyst* (Iedema and Carroll, 2011). The clinalyst is an outsider person who comes in with a fairly well-defined aim and facilitates reflexivity using video footage to achieve this aim. If you are an 'outsider' researcher taking a clinalyst stance, you will consult clinicians about what kinds of footage they want to view, but you might remain largely in control of choosing clips and will likely facilitate reflexive discussions by asking questions to encourage discussion about predetermined issues (Iedema and Carroll, 2011). Vignette 5.1 provides an example.

Another way of thinking about collaboration can be described as planned obsolescence. Here, your strategy is not just to conduct VRE but also to hand the VRE process over to local practitioners, so that they are enabled to do it themselves. If you are a researcher facilitating planned obsolescence, you might provide advice and support to clinicians about how they can design, promote and facilitate reflexive sessions towards their own desired outcomes (Mesman, 2015). Vignettes 5.2 and 5.3 provide examples of this. In Vignette 5.2, the researcher initially worked closely with clinicians to co-create footage

---

Vignette 5.1   A study deploying 'the clinalyst'

Title of project	Anchoring healthcare improvement to positive learning
Researchers, institution	R. Iedema, D. Long, B. Lee (University of New South Wales, Sydney, New South Wales, Australia)
Funder	Australian Research Council
Aims of study	Involve front-line clinicians in exploring their practice with the aim of enabling them to learn about how to improve their own practices and relationships
Participants	A multidisciplinary team including medical, nursing and allied health professionals
Field site	A high-performing spinal unit in a major metropolitan teaching hospital
Collaborating with clinicians to choose footage	The researcher worked closely with clinical co-researchers to select themes and footage, as well as to set up the infrastructure for communication in the first stage of the project.
Publications	Iedema et al. (2006), Long et al. (2006), Iedema et al. (2009b)

Vignette 5.2	A study aiming for researcher obsolescence
Title of project	Safety from a new angle: exnovation and VRE on the NICU
Researchers, institution	J. Mesman (Maastricht University, Maastricht, The Netherlands)
Aims of study	Implement the VRE methodology as a structural aspect of the NICU
	Identify good practices of infection prevention
Participants	All clinicians on the NICU participated in the VRE reflectivity meetings. Four clinicians were trained as members of the VRE working group to enable them to use the method independent of a researcher for practice improvement
Field site	The 'planned obsolescence' team training took place on the intensive care for newborns of the Maastricht University Medical Centre in the Netherlands
Collaborating with clinicians to choose footage	The researcher worked closely with clinical co-researchers to select themes and footage, as well as to set up the infrastructure for communication in the first stage of the project. While the training progressed, the researcher became gradually less involved
Publications	Carroll and Mesman (2018), Mesman (2007), Mesman (2015)

and to decide on themes and clips for each session. The clinicians' investment in the project resulted in them being able to conduct VRE independent of the researcher.

In Vignette 5.3, the researchers invited study participants to determine what they saw as brilliant examples of end-of-life care. In this sense, the study was driven by participating clinicians.

Third, your study may be openly 'emotion-driven'. This is what Carroll and Mesman (2018) refer to as 'affect-as-method'. If you are using VRE in an 'affect-as-method' mode, you may proceed unprogrammatically by being fully oriented towards the concerns of your participants. This mode leaves the direction of your engagement open until issues present themselves that take on special significance and momentum for your participants (Iedema and Carroll, 2015). Vignette 5.4 exemplifies this.

In practice, you may mobilize each of these three modes to various degrees depending on how reliant participants want to be on your guidance and facilitation ('clinalyst'), how keen they are to practise VRE on processes and at a pace of their choosing ('obsolescence') or how happy participants are to keep your relationship with them open-ended and explore practice without preset agenda ('affect-as-method').

Vignette 5.3 A study capturing 'Brilliance' in evidence-based palliative care

Title of project	Brilliance in evidence-based palliative care
Researchers, institutions	A. Dadich, M. Hodgins (Western Sydney University, Sydney, New South Wales, Australia), A. Collier (University of Auckland, Auckland, New Zealand)
	Other investigators: M. Agar, J. Harlum, P. Waldon, T. Smeal (New South Wales)
	Other investigators: G. Crawford (South Australia)
	Co-researchers: K. Womsley, S. Kang, V. Weller (New South Wales)
	Co-researchers: C. Jeffs, C. Farrow, P. Houthuysen (South Australia)
Funders	New South Wales (Agency for Clinical Innovation and University of Western Sydney)
	South Australia (Modbury Hospital Foundation and Flinders University)
Aims of study	To promote brilliance in evidence-based palliative care
	Objectives:
	1. Identify brilliant exemplars of evidence-based palliative care in community settings
	2. Examine and critique associated effects
	3. Determine the conditions required for and/or associated with brilliance in evidence-based palliative care
	4. Develop a framework clarifying the conditions in which evidence-based palliative care that is brilliant is likely to flourish in community settings
Participants	Multidisciplinary team members of a community palliative care team (including non-clinical staff) and patients and family carers under their care
Field site	Outer metropolitan community palliative care teams in two states of Australia (New South Wales and South Australia) field-work took place in peoples' homes, in clinicians' vehicles, as well as at the teams' office base.
Collaborating with clinicians to choose footage	The researchers worked closely with clinical co-researchers in both states to collect data, review footage and make decisions about what to show back to other clinical colleagues. The level of engagement and confidence of co-researchers increased as the study progressed. Their investment in the project was, to a large extent, a result of focusing on strengths rather than gaps in care delivery
Publications	Dadich et al. (2018), Collier et al. (accepted)
Acknowledgements	The authors acknowledge all the brilliant co-researchers, clinicians, patients and carers who participated in the project

	Vignette 5.4 A study guided by affect
Title of project	The use of donor milk in Australian and American neonatal intensive care units
Researchers, institution	K. Carroll (Australian National University, Acton, Canberra, Australia)
Aims of study	To understand how donor milk was positioned relative to other types of infant feeding (such as a mother's own milk and artificial formula) in the broader context where donor milk is now recognized as a better food compared to formula when a mother's own milk is unavailable
Participants	Neonatal intensive care doctors, nurses, dieticians and social workers
Field site	Australian and American neonatal intensive care units
Collaborating with clinicians to choose footage	This is how Carroll describes the way her collaboration unfolded: 'As I watched the staff trying to maximise the scarce [and expensive] donor breastmilk and the last few millilitres of one mother's own breastmilk, I, the videographer and researcher, became affected by the situation and felt "moved to act." ... I realised that the difficulty faced by the neonatal clinicians, the family and the infant was not limited to this one case. ... I ... decided to act ... using the video footage to see what the clinicians themselves would say were they to see themselves acting within and facing the consequences of this dilemma. In preparation, I edited a short clip portraying the case and associated clinical discussions, and then showed it to the medical staff and clinical team. In addition to the video clip, I also presented cost analysis data on feeding infants donor milk ... As the clinicians watched the footage of the prescribing doctor dealing with the mother and the sick baby, they witnessed the contradiction between their espoused values (care for people, prescribe donor breast milk), their donor milk policies, and their *in situ* actions. What they saw went against "the organisation that they wanted to be".'
Publications	Carroll and Herrmann (2013), Carroll (2014), Iedema and Carroll (2015)

These three modes of collaboration highlight three different dimensions of VRE. The clinalyst underscores VRE's concern to have a practical and tangible effect. The obsolescence strategy underscores VRE's democratic, educational and learning priorities, as it entrusts practitioners and patients with adopting this method for their own betterment, on their own terms. For its part, affect-as-method underscores the significance of *affect* as the basis of research (Iedema and

Carroll, 2015), framing the relationship between the researcher and the practitioner/patient as in the first and last instances an emotional one, and thereby turning the values commonly associated with research on their head. That is, to accommodate the conditions of complexity, objectivity, distance and rigour become recast as subjective involvement, closeness and flexibility (Carroll and Mesman, 2018).

Finally, let us consider the issues that arise when collaborating with patients and families. Chapter 1 examined how the theoretical and philosophical underpinnings of VRE have, to a large extent, shaped how we have come to appreciate whose knowledge counts in healthcare practice, research and policy. Although most VRE research to date has focused on clinicians, there are increasing numbers of studies engaging patients and families in video-reflexivity (Collier et al., 2015; Wyer et al., 2015; Collier et al., 2016; McLeod et al., 2016; McLeod, 2017; Wyer et al., 2017). Patients and their families in these studies have been involved in scrutinizing videoed care for patient safety communication and risks, as well as choosing footage that will be shown back to the clinicians who care for them. Collier and Wyer (2016) explore the particular potentials and challenges of conducting reflexive sessions with patients and their families including creating safe spaces for patients to voice their healthcare concerns and for clinicians to 'hear' patients' perspectives on the care they receive. They conclude that iterative and multi-layered researcher reflexivity in the field is critical to the progress and success of studies seeking to use VRE with patients.

Other ways of conducting collaborative reflexive sessions with both patients and clinicians have been explored too. For example, reflexive sessions have been trialled where a researcher, a patient and a clinician viewed footage together (Wyer, 2017). This produced distinctive and productive conversations about patient safety risks and has led to the development of a study by Wyer, Hor, Gilbert and other collaborators that commenced in early 2018, in a renal unit at a large metropolitan hospital in Sydney. VRE is used in this study to improve clinician–patient communication around health-care-associated infection screening and identification. Along with Dadich and Hodgins and their co-researcher clinical colleagues, Collier has recently also facilitated reflexive sessions in people's homes involving patients and their families after a person has died (Hodgins et al., 2016; Dadich et al., 2018).

Mesman has conducted reflexive sessions with parents-to-be, midwives and obstetricians. The nuanced feedback she obtained from the participating parents revealed informal competences on the part of the obstetricians and midwives undergirding their communication and collaboration with parents (to be) (Korstjens et al., 2018). Consideration has also been given to facilitating video-reflexive sessions with groups of patients (without clinicians) to provide opportunities for them to draw on their shared intelligence and increase their potential for adapting their (health) behaviours (Wadnerkar et al., 2011).

5.2.3 Reflexivity

At the beginning of this chapter, we distinguished between reflection and reflexivity. We defined reflection as a private activity focusing on individuals' past. Reflexivity was defined as a shared deliberative process enabling participants to apprehend and frame their selves, practices and circumstances in new ways (Iedema, 2011). The point of reflexivity is not principally to gain more or better knowledge about things that have occurred, but to create the possibility for new understandings, new perspectives, new identities and new social futures.

As we have discussed thus far, watching back footage of oneself and others and/or listening to accounts of care provides people the opportunity to review what they do, how they do it and with whom. This confronts them with aspects of their work and context in a novel way. Seeing themselves at work is novel, and seeing that work from an unexpected angle is also novel. In an earlier paper, using an idea of MacDougall (2006), we argued that seeing yourself on screen at once distances you from what is shown and it brings things closer (Carroll et al., 2008). This too will be novel: realizing that what is shown represents us, and at the same time making that which has always appeared so familiar distant and strange.

5.2.4 Reflexive meetings and care

Not surprisingly, people can be anxious initially about what they are about to see. The novelty of seeing themselves on screen usually produces a multitude of cognitive and emotional responses. For this reason, we need to tread cautiously. Processing all the new information that becomes available through watching the footage can be exciting, but it can also be taxing. For example, one of the authors showed back a clip of a nurse and physician travelling in the car while discussing the complexities of care and their decision-making concerning the patient and family they had just visited. What might easily have been deemed "relatively mundane" by those watching turned out to be highly significant. The footage portrayed the busyness of clinicians driving through traffic and discussing cases. When shown to the team, the footage elicited discussion about why community staff might be so tired at the end of a day. The discussion proceeded to touch on strategies for self-care. The discussion also touched on how the team might help other clinicians to become better at recognizing when people are dying.

We have found that showing clips can have a considerable emotional impact on those watching them. People express surprise, shame, a determination to address things and pride or disappointment in what they see. Affect therefore plays a prominent role in VRE. Even if we position ourselves primarily as a clinalyst, or as someone intending to hand the video process over to practitioners themselves, we still have to monitor people's emotional responses to the videoing, the footage used for feedback and the things that are said. In fact, our view is that affect permeates how we do research generally, researchers' claims about enacting objectivity, rigour and distance notwithstanding. Affect is a critical resource for participative research such as VRE (Iedema and Carroll, 2015). This last statement is not a gratuitous nicety. We prize affect because it is integral to the quality and safety of care, and it modulates how we attend to the well-being of others and ourselves (Iedema et al., 2009a).

Capitalizing on how vision foregrounds affect, VRE enables, encourages and requires participants to become vulnerable in order to learn and change. Viewing and reflecting on footage asks that people put at risk 'not just specific aspects of their behaviour [...] but their personal identity and, thereby, their social and organisational relationships' (Iedema, 2011: i84–i85). It is therefore of utmost importance to establish and maintain a safe space where people can be vulnerable. This requires a lot of preparation and care. VRE facilitators must be sensitive and adaptive to the context and politics of the research space during videoing, editing and conducting research relationships. It is arguably even more important for facilitators of reflexive sessions to be constantly aware of, and responsive to, participants' reactions and dynamics during reflexive sessions. This is the case whether you have an informal session around the laptop in the tea room with 3 people, or 25 people in a large meeting room with a projector and screen.

In Chapter 2, we described a 'situational ethics' approach to VRE and the need for such an approach to the planning and running of video-reflexive sessions. We have tended towards an ethically conservative approach in deciding which clips to show, being mindful of the content of those clips as well as the actors who feature in them. Our practice has been to provide opportunities for those represented to see the clip(s) in question and to seek consent from them prior to the clip(s) being shown to larger audiences.

We are also mindful that some participants may want to be present when the clip is shown, while others may choose not to. Some participants may be happy for the clip to be shown but prefer not to see it prior. For example, in one VRE study, patients with a life-limiting illness were keen for clinicians to see their accounts of care but most preferred not to watch the footage themselves (Collier, 2013). A participant may be comfortable with and consent to a clip being shown to their nurse peers but prefer not to have their manager see it. Clinicians in a large group video-reflexive session discussed in Vignette 5.3 requested that the viewing order be changed if clips were to be shown in a reflexive session with senior management.

Furthermore, in deciding which clips to show, we have avoided showing clips that are particularly controversial or that demonstrate what could be viewed as negative. For example, in one study, patients brought up issues of concern that they wanted to communicate to nursing staff. Some of the patients' comments were quite critical and might have been quite confronting for the nurses. Despite feeling strongly that patients should drive the messages conveyed, the researcher discussed (but did not insist on) the options other than showing the identifiable video with the patient for relaying the message; for example, showing the patient's concern in the form of an anonymized quote. There were several reasons for doing the latter, including maintaining therapeutic patient/nurse relationships as well as maintaining research relationships with the nurses that would keep them open to seeing and hearing the experiences and concerns of patients under their care (Collier and Wyer, 2016).

The Brilliance study (Vignette 5.3) was perhaps an exception to this where the study was framed within Positive Organisational Scholarship (POS), and the explicit aim of the study was to identify 'brilliant' exemplars of care (Dadich et al., 2016, 2018). Brilliant practice however is very much in the eye of the beholder, and even in this study, the POS framing did not mean that researchers did not use clips that warranted questions being asked about the practice shown.

It bears repeating at this point that no decision you make about these issues will be neutral and value-free. What one person may view as harmless or controversial is not necessarily seen so by another and vice versa. Nevertheless, it may sometimes be evident that a clip is seen as embarrassing or offensive to a particular individual and/or individuals. This is why it is critical to check clips beforehand with insider participants. Facilitators will need to have strategies ready to deal with possible negative emotions arising among participants. As we detail in Chapter 6, reiterating the reason for your VRE study and acknowledging the courage and generosity of those who have allowed their footage to be used for learning can assist in alleviating people's concerns. At all times, explain the ground rules that act as a foundation for creating and maintaining a safe reflexive space. These ground rules include (among other things) maintaining mutual respect and avoiding personal blame.

Our experience has taught us that it is helpful to be aware of power dynamics when bringing different groups together for reflexive sessions: managers and clinicians, junior staff together with senior staff, one particular discipline with another, and patients and clinicians. You may or may not be aware of the political dynamics or power relations in a clinical environment or the history of these. You could be walking into a minefield if you have brought the occupational therapists together with the physiotherapists to watch footage, and you are not aware that they have been involved in a significant dispute over the blurring of their roles for the past 2 years. Occasionally, you may even have to curtail or abandon a session. If, for example, five managers turn up to a session with only two junior nurses, the power dynamic in the session may simply be too overwhelming for those involved.

Attention to these power dynamics may be of particular relevance if you are involving patients and families in VRE. You will need to think carefully about bringing together patients with clinicians. What implications might this have again in terms of power dynamics, and most critically perhaps, how might doing so affect a person's ongoing care? We will return to consider these issues later when we discuss some of the occasions when video-reflexive sessions have not gone so well. Table 5.1 summarizes the above discussion thus far.

Table 5.1 Planning reflexive sessions

Theoretical principles	What clips to show	How to guide the reflexive discussion
1. Exnovation	The clips show a variety and range of behaviours instantiating a practice	Invite participants to respond to and explain what is happening
2. Collaboration	The clips show what participants are interested in and what they feel strongly about	Invite participants to participate in and lead the discussion as experts

(Continued)

Table 5.1 (*Continued*) Planning reflexive sessions

Theoretical principles	What clips to show	How to guide the reflexive discussion
3. Reflexivity	The clips create disruptions in people's understanding of and perspective on their practice and behaviour	Question simple explanations and invite alternative accounts; ask questions rather than making statements; the tipping point happens when participants start asking themselves and each other questions
4. Care	The clips have been subjected to consent and careful vetting before being shown to team members. The social/political implications of showing particular clips have been thought through, and participants' comfort levels have been carefully tested and are constantly monitored	Make sure you have an acute sense of how people position themselves in the reflexive meetings: sense whether they are overly critical of themselves or of others, and divert the discussion away from blame and guilt; monitor the group's dynamics and aim to involve everyone by inviting silent attendees to comment or respond and by directing the discussion away from overly vocal ones; carefully monitor how people deal with sensitive issues and who gets the last say about them; highlight strengths and only gently nudge people towards considering any shortcomings (if they haven't called attention to those already); the mood of the meeting needs to be 'wow, what can we do with this', and not 'gosh, how terrible are we/they'; be aware of those who hold up the rules that should have been followed but weren't and 'what should have been done instead', and see if you can guide the discussion towards problematizing the rules, and towards the group/team agreeing on what are *their* rules

5.3 REFLEXIVE SESSIONS: PRACTICAL CONSIDERATIONS

We now turn to some of the practicalities you may want to consider when planning video-reflexive sessions.

5.3.1 Preparing for reflexive sessions – Main purpose

A key consideration in conducting a video-reflexive session is the purpose of the session and how this affects the way you facilitate the session. Is your purpose that of a clinalyst, where the video-reflexive session aims to illuminate the specific aspects of practice for improving that practice? Or do you want the session to be steered by the practitioners or the patients? Or are you aiming to explore issues or tensions to understand better how practitioners and patients feel about them? The answers to these questions have implications for how you might prepare and plan your session, who will facilitate it and who will be invited and by whom. These decisions, of course, are not solely practical ones but have implications for group and power dynamics as well as for ongoing relationships with participants.

If the video-reflexive session is taking place in the context of a targeted research question, the session is likely to be framed with a focus on progressing the discussion towards practical solutions or to gain insights regarding quite specific phenomena. If your aim is practitioner/patient learning, you are more likely to spend time on creating opportunities for people to appreciate the developmental potential of video feedback. If your aim is to target tensions, conflicts, sentiments and the like, you will most likely be very concerned to know and keep track of people's responses and reactions to the footage and to one another's comments. This is not to limit VRE to addressing one or the other of the above, because VRE has the capacity to straddle them all. Rather, we suggest that you consider the aim and purpose of any particular session carefully in advance with a view to sketching out likely scenarios, and think through how to manage them in case they arise.

5.3.2 How many reflexive sessions do you need and when should they take place?

There is no prescription for the number of structured reflexive sessions required for any particular VRE project. However, you can plan for a number of sessions, and depending on the outcomes of these, plan for more. Figure 5.1 is an example showing a 3-month VRE research project, where reflexive sessions were planned at 4, 7 and 10 weeks with a final feedback session in the 12th week. This plan allowed plenty of time to develop relationships and co-create video footage with participants before the first reflexive session took place. It also left room for extra structured sessions to be held if the participants wished to explore particular themes in more depth.

If you are conducting a project in your own workplace and already have good working relationships with your colleagues, they may be ready to commence

Timeline (March to May)											
Month 1				Month 2				Month 3			
Week 1	2	3	4	5	6	7	8	9	10	11	12
Interviews; Observations; Videoing			Reflexive session/s	Videoing; Interviews		Reflexive session/s		Videoing; Interviews	Reflexive session/s	Analysis	Final feedback session
Ongoing video-editing, analysis and transcription of interviews and reflexive sessions											

Figure 5.1 A 3-month VRE research project.

Timeline (August to September)							
Month 1				Month 2			
Week 1	2	3	4	5	6	7	8
Interviews; Observations; Videoing	Reflexive session/s	Videoing; Interviews	Videoing; Reflexive sessions	Videoing; Reflexive sessions	Videoing; Reflexive sessions	Videoing; Reflexive sessions	Final feedback session
Ongoing video-editing and analysis							

Figure 5.2 A 2-month clinician-led VRE research project.

videoing immediately, and you may not need to wait so long for your first and subsequent reflexive sessions (see Figure 5.2).

Organizing structured video-reflexive sessions with clinicians can sometimes present challenges however. First, and for obvious reasons, gathering together a group of busy healthcare staff (be they doctors, nurses, allied health, administrative or managerial staff) in the same space and at the same time, when their focus is on the minute-to-minute and day-to-day core business of healthcare work, can pose a significant challenge. Second, in accordance with guiding principle 2 (collaboration), the underpinning *modus operandi* of doing VRE is to work with healthcare staff and others who have the right to be involved in everything we do. This requires working out, with those staff in a particular context, what is going to be most feasible for them in terms of when, where and with whom video-reflexive sessions can occur.

While planning group reflexive sessions is discussed in Chapter 6, let us briefly comment on it here. Planning group reflexive sessions to take place within an already existing structure, for example, during a regular team meeting or an in-service session, is usually a good way to ensure that people are able to attend. Additionally, if your aim is 'planned obsolescence', then integrating sessions into already existing structures might increase the likelihood that video-reflexivity is embedded in those structures as a 'normal' part of everyday practice. Thus, finding out when meetings and staff forums are held can be useful, as well as who is responsible for organizing them and/or who the key people are who might help you promote the session. For example, in the study described in Vignette 5.3, reflexive sessions were held in the weekly education time slot. The advantage of doing so was that most staff regularly attended this weekly meeting and used it as a time to 'stop' and consider their practice. Thus, reflection at this time was already a feature of their work. Another advantage was that the meeting was held in a large room with audio–visual facilities that could be used for the video-reflexive activities.

5.3.3 Who should attend structured reflexive sessions and how will you invite them?

Who should attend a particular session depends very much on what you and the participants hope to achieve during the session. For example, if the aim of the session is to make sense of a practice through the perspectives of members of different disciplines, then you will likely invite as many members as possible from these different disciplines. Alternatively, you may want to start first with sessions that give space for single disciplines to view footage and explore a practice before bringing everyone together to share their experiences and ideas. If the aim of the session is to make decisions about practice change, for example, during a final feedback session (see Section 6.8), you will want to negotiate with managers and other decision makers to ensure they can be present.

If you are an external researcher, you may not be the person best placed to make decisions about who should attend meetings. Instead, you may need to liaise with ward champions to decide when it is best to bring managers and clinicians together for a specific purpose. Ward nurses might have a creative practice idea in response to footage but need the ward managers' understanding of why and how their solution might be put into practice. Conversely, a group of managers may think they've come up with a critical solution, but that solution may be completely unworkable in practice from the perspective of front-line clinicians or patients.

As suggested earlier, you should ensure that those featured in the clips that will be shown at the session are given the opportunity to attend if they wish (or to be made aware that their clip will be shown if they do not wish to attend). This will also impact when the session can be held, as you may need to find a time when those in the footage can actually be present. This can be particularly difficult when staff is on rotating rosters. Make sure you have telephone numbers or other reliable forms of contact details for those who have been videoed, so you can contact them to make sure they will be available when sessions are taking place and to obtain ongoing consent to use their footage.

Ensuring that the necessary people are invited to a session requires finding out the best communication channels to reach them. Utilize your project champion(s) to find out this information. How is information commonly passed on to staff? Where do they find out about events? Do staff have access to email and are they likely to read it? Does the ward have a communication book? Is a poster in the tea room or at the workstation likely to be noticed (see Figure 5.3)? Is there a staff mail system by which you can send or drop a hard copy invitation? Can you speak to teams of doctors face-to-face before their morning meetings?

5.3.4 What clips will you show? How many?

We have already described earlier in this chapter how the guiding principles can help you to choose what kinds of clips you might show in your reflexive session (see Table 5.1). For most 30–60-min sessions, we find it useful to have a bank of

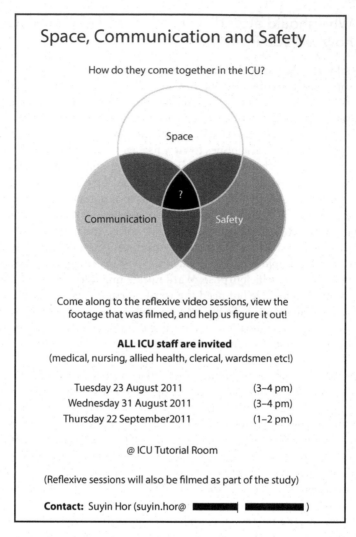

Figure 5.3 Advertising poster. (Image courtesy of Su-yin Hor.)

five or six clips ready to use. This allows for flexibility. Should the discussion go off on an unexpected tangent, you will be able to adapt to the session, including which clips you show in relation to the ensuing dialogue. We should perhaps also mention here that our experience is often one of nervous anticipation as we approach a video-reflexive session. Will participants find selected clips relevant and meaningful? Will anyone respond?

We have come to appreciate that these thoughts and feelings are part and parcel of the uncertainty inherent in engaging with VRE and facilitating video-reflexive sessions (Carroll, 2009). Your willingness and ability to adapt according to how a session unfolds therefore are necessary pre-requisites of video-reflexive sessions. Preparing as much as possible however does go some way to providing a counterbalance to the feeling of uncertainty. While participants may also be uncertain about what will happen, our experience is usually that even the most mundane of clips can engender much response. For this reason, we have found that confidence in the process, and not more than four to five short (i.e. 1–3-min) clips are usually sufficient to elicit discussion for a typical hour-long session.

5.3.5 What equipment will you need?

Paying attention to technical issues in advance is important, so you can concentrate on the content of your reflexive session. We have sometimes found ourselves in situations where we have carefully edited all of our clips and have gone to great effort to ensure participants are attending, only to find that the room we booked didn't have the necessary audio–visual equipment, or our clips were in a format not read by the software on the computer in the presentation room. Doing a trial run is always necessary to make sure that your session will run without technical hitches. Table 5.2 provides several other suggestions for consideration.

Table 5.2 Equipment

Equipment you might need	Issues to consider
Laptop or desktop computer	**Large group reflexive sessions**
	Can you connect to a projector?
	If using your own laptop, ensure you have correct adaptors for connecting to the facility projector.
	If using a facility's computer equipment, check that you're able to transfer your presentation files and that your movie files are in the correct format for playing on the available system.
	Small group reflexive sessions
	Is your laptop screen large enough for everyone in the group to see?
	If you are using a facility desktop computer, follow the above advice regarding hard drive/USB and movie files.
Projector	If people cannot see the footage, they can quickly lose interest.
	For groups greater than four or five, large-scale projection of footage assists with better engagement. Check that your reflexive space has a projector, and if not, locate one you can use. Buying your own portable projector may be a useful investment.
Adaptor cables	As suggested above, carrying a variety of laptop-to-projector adaptor cables is wise. If possible, check the requirements in advance.

(Continued)

Table 5.2 (*Continued*) Equipment

Equipment you might need	Issues to consider
Screen or wall space for projection	In rooms not set up for presentations (e.g. staff tea rooms), you may find it hard to access clear space for projection. Clear wall space in advance (with permission from appropriate staff) and check that your projection is adequate beforehand.
Speakers	If you are relying on sound, check that whatever system you are using provides audio loud enough for participants to hear. Having a set of speakers that can connect to your computer can be helpful.
Video camera(s)	If you want to video the reflexive session, you will need to bring your camera(s) and make sure the batteries are charged
Tripod	A video camera tripod can be useful for positioning your video camera so as to capture the reflexive session in frame.
Power leads/ power board	Bring power leads for laptops, cameras, speakers and/or projector where appropriate. A power board can be useful for rooms with few power sources.
Spare batteries	Make sure you have spare, charged batteries for your video camera, if available.
Audio recorders	Audio recorders are useful: 1. In large group sessions – for placing in a few sites around the room so as to capture all the voices and enabling easier transcription of discussions. 2. As backup if members of the group would rather not be video-recorded or the session takes place in a public area where it is not appropriate or feasible to video-record.
Consent forms Information handouts Pens	Have consent forms and handouts ready for those who have not yet attended an information session or who have not signed consent
Catering	Snacks are always appreciated!

5.3.6 Preparing the space

5.3.6.1 SEATING

It can be worth thinking about how to arrange seating at reflexive sessions. We have found that arranging seats in a semicircle (rather than in rows) or around a table can encourage more inclusive discussion. Having people seated around a table also means you can make handouts and consent forms accessible as well as any catering supplies. We have also found that moving all the chairs up to the front of the room can discourage people from congregating at the back of the room and not participating in discussions. Make sure everyone can see the screen.

5.3.6.2 RECORDING THE SESSION

If you plan to video record the session for analysis later, think about where to best place your camera(s). Recording from the front of the room results in footage that clearly allows you to identify who is speaking when you are watching or analyzing footage (see Figure 5.4). Videoing from behind can provide a good view of the facilitator, the screen and the participants. This can be helpful in understanding the context of the discussion as you can see what aspects of the footage participants are referring to (see Figure 5.5). Sometimes, it is possible to video from directly behind the facilitator, and this can give a view of the facilitator, the computer screen that they are looking at and the participants beyond (see Figure 5.6). Having someone to assist you with monitoring equipment and making sure that they are recording throughout the session can be useful. A tripod with tilt options can also be useful for securing your video camera in a stable position that will successfully capture the session in its entirety.

As suggested in Table 5.2, placing one (or two) audio recorder(s) around the room maximizes your chances of obtaining a clear recording of all the participants' contributions to the discussion, especially if your video camera microphones are not high quality.

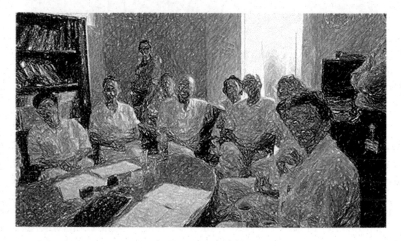

Figure 5.4 Videoing from the front of the room results in footage that clearly allows you to identify who is speaking when you are watching or analyzing footage. (Image courtesy of Jessica Mesman.)

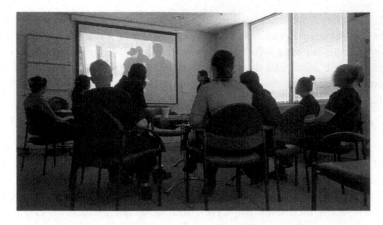

Figure 5.5 Videoing reflexive session from behind allows you to see screen and participants. (Photo courtesy of Su-yin Hor, Sydney, Australia and Mary Wyer.)

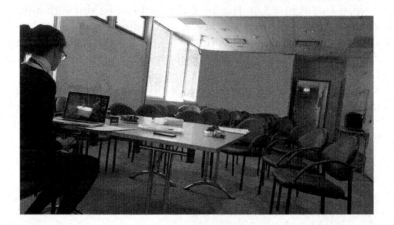

Figure 5.6 Video footage shot from directly behind the facilitator with a view of the computer screen and of the room set up for participants. (Photo courtesy of Su-yin Hor and Mary Wyer.)

5.4 CONCLUSION

This chapter has set out the general principles for preparing for and planning reflexive meetings. Critical issues here were thinking through the kinds of clips you may want to show, and the process of checking these clips with insider-collaborators to ensure you have not missed anything sensitive or embarrassing. Practical considerations were raised, such as preparing the room where the session is held and thinking through what may happen given your likely audience. Chapter 6 delves into the running of reflexive meetings, paying specific attention to the practical dimensions of managing creative and volatile discussions.

REFERENCES

Bennett T, Dodsworth F, Noble G, et al. (2013) Habit and habituation: Governance and the social. *Body & Society* 19: 3–29.

Carroll K. (2009) Outsider, insider, alongsider: Examining reflexivity in hospital-based video research. *International Journal of Multiple Research Approaches* 3: 246–263.

Carroll K. (2014) Body dirt or liquid gold? How the safety of donor human milk is constructed for use in neonatal intensive care. *Social Studies of Science* 44: 466–485.

Carroll K and Herrmann K. (2013) The cost of using donor human milk in the NICU to achieve exclusively human milk feeding through 32 weeks post-menstrual age. *Breastfeeding Medicine* 8: 286–290.

Carroll K, Iedema R and Kerridge R. (2008) Reshaping ICU ward round practices using video reflexive ethnography. *Qualitative Health Research* 18: 380–390.

Carroll K and Mesman J. (2018) Multiple researcher roles in video-reflexive ethnography. *Qualitatve Health Research*. 28(7): 1145–56.

Collier A. (2013) Deleuzians of patient safety: A video reflexive ethnography of end-of-life care. PhD Thesis. Sydney: Faculty of Arts and Social Sciences, University of Techology.

Collier A, Hodgins M, Crawford G, et al. (accepted) What does it take to deliver brilliant home-based palliative care? Using positive organisational scholarship and video reflexive ethnography to explore the complexities of palliative care at home. *Palliative Medicine*.

Collier A, Phillips J and Iedema R. (2015) The meaning of home at the end of life: A video-reflexive ethnography study. *Palliative Medicine* 29: 695–702.

Collier A, Sorensen R and Iedema R. (2016) Patients' and families' perspectives of patient safety at the end of life: A video-reflexive ethnography study. *International Journal for Quality in Health Care* 28: 66–73.

Collier A and Wyer M. (2016) Researching reflexively with patients and families: Two studies using video-reflexive ethnography to collaborate with patients and families in patient safety research. *Qualitative Health Research* 26: 979–993.

Dadich A, Collier A and Hodgins M. (2018) Using POSH VRE to examine positive deviance to new public management in healthcare. *Qualitative Health Research* 28(8): 1203–1216.

Dadich A, Hodgins M and Collier A. (2016) Video reflexive ethnography: A creative approach to understand and promote brilliant organisational experiences. In: *ACSPRI (Australian Consortium for Social and Political Research Incorporated) Social Science Methodology Conference.* University of Sydney, Australia, July.

Dewey J. (1922) *Human Nature and Conduct: An Introduction to Social Psychology.* New York: H. Holt & Company.

Greatbatch D, Murphy E and Dingwall R. (2001) Evaluating medical information systems: Ethnomethodological and interactionist approaches. *Health Services Management Research* 14: 181–191.

Grosz E. (2013) Habit today: Ravaisson, Bergson, Deleuze and us. *Body & Society* 19: 217–239.

Hodgins M, Dadich A and Collier A. (2016) Negotiating access and undertaking video reflexive ethnography in community-based palliative care. In: *ACSPRI (Australian Consortium for Social and Political Research Incorporated) Social Science Methodology Conference.* University of Sydney, Australia, July.

Iedema R. (2011) Creating safety by strengthening clinicians' capacity for reflexivity. *BMJ Quality and Safety* 20: S83–S86.

Iedema R and Carroll K. (2011) The clinalyst: Institutionalizing reflexive space to realize safety and flexible systematization in health care. *Journal of Organizational Change Management* 24: 175–190.

Iedema R and Carroll K. (2015) Research as affect-sphere: Towards spherogenics. *Emotion Review* 7: 1–7.

Iedema R, Long D, Forsyth R, et al. (2006) Visibilizing clinical work: Video ethnography in the contemporary hospital. *Health Sociology Review* 15: 156–168.

Iedema R, Jorm C and Lum M. (2009a) Affect is central to patient safety: The horror stories of young anaesthetists. *Social Science & Medicine* 69: 1750–1756.

Iedema R, Merrick E, Rajbhandari D, et al. (2009b) Viewing the taken-for-granted from under a different aspect: A video-based method in pursuit of patient safety. *International Journal for Multiple Research Approaches* 3: 290–301.

Iedema R, Mesman J and Carroll K. (2013) *Visualising Health Care Practice Improvement: Innovation from Within.* London: Radcliffe.

Korstjens I, Mesman J, van Helmond I, et al. (2018) *Exnovating for better birth: An investigation of the collaborative practices in Dutch maternity care.* Available at: www.av-m.nl/midwifery-science/studies/exnovating-for-better-birth

Long D, Forsyth R, Carroll K, et al. (2006) The (im)possibility of clinical democracy. *Health Sociology Review* 15: 506–519.

MacDougall D. (2006) *The Corporeal Image: Film, Ethnography and the Senses.* Princeton, NJ: Princeton University Press.

McLeod H. (2017) Respect and shared decision making in the clinical encounter: A video-reflexive ethnography. PhD Thesis. University of Minnesota.

McLeod H, Bywaters D, Collier A, et al. (2016) The patient revolution and video-reflexive ethnography. In: *ACSPRI Social Science Methodology Conference.* University of Sydney, 19–22 July.

Mesman J. (2007) Disturbing observations as a basis for collaborative research. *Science as Culture* 16: 281–295.

Mesman J. (2011) Resources of strength: An exnovation of hidden competences to preserve patient safety. In: Rowley E and Waring J (eds) A *Sociocultural Perspective on Patient Safety.* Farnham: Ashgate.

Mesman J. (2015) Boundary spanning engagement on the neonatal ward: Reflections on a collaborative entanglement between clinicians and a researcher. In: Penders B, Vermeulen N, and Parker J (eds) *Collaboration across Health Research and Medical Care.* Farnham: Ashgate, 171–194.

Nilsen P, Roback K, Brostrom A, et al. (2012) Creatures of habit: Accounting for the role of habit in implementation research on clinical behaviour change. *Implementation Science* 7(1): 1–6.

Shusterman R. (2008) *Body Consciousness: A Philosophy of Mindfulness and Somaesthetics*. Cambridge: Cambridge University Press.

Sloterdijk P. (2013) *You Must Change Your Life*. Cambridge: Polity Press.

Wadnerkar MB, Pirinen T, Haines-Bazrafshan R, et al. (2011) A single case study of a family-centred intervention with a young girl with cerebral palsy who is a multimodal communicator. *Child: Care, Health and Development.* 38(1), 87–97.

Wittgenstein L. (1953) *Philosophical Investigations*. Oxford: Blackwell.

Wyer M. (2017) Integrating patients' experiences, understandings and enactments of infection prevention and control into clinicians' everyday care: A video-reflexive ethnographic exploratory intervention. University of Tasmania.

Wyer M, Iedema R, Hor S, et al. (2017) Patient involvement can affect clinicians' perspectives and practices of infection prevention and control: A 'post-qualitative' study using video-reflexive ethnography. *International Journal of Qualitative Research Methods* 16: 1–10.

Wyer M, Jackson D, Iedema R, et al. (2015) Involving patients in understanding hospital infection control using visual methods. *Journal of Clinical Nursing.* 24(11–12): 1718–1729.

6

Conducting reflexive sessions

6.1 INTRODUCTION

This chapter discusses the facilitation of reflexive sessions. As the previous chapters have made clear, reflexive sessions form a critical component of the overall video-reflexive ethnography (VRE) process. Their dynamics are defining the progress of your project, and their outcomes are defining your project's success. In this chapter, we discuss different ways of facilitating reflexive sessions, and we provide examples from our work to illustrate our points. We then move on to describe what may be said during the sessions and in what ways these sessions are – or can be – unique. We offer some reflections on what it means to enact researcher reflexivity, and we conclude the chapter with some accounts of things going wrong – as they sometimes do!

6.2 DIFFERENT APPROACHES TO RUNNING REFLEXIVE SESSIONS

Running reflexive sessions is not always easy. Even when sessions have been planned and booked in advance, it can still be a challenge to bring practitioners and/or patients together in the same room at the same time and get (and sustain) their attention. While community settings may offer opportunities for people to gather, in the often frenetic setting of the acute hospital it may be impossible for people to 'gather' in one place for a group session, especially when you are trying to gather participants from different disciplines who rarely participate in shared meetings. In some situations, staff can become anxious if they are asked to be away from their patients and their work for too long.

In some circumstances, you may need to take the session to your participants. This may mean finding moments during quiet times during the day, on the ward or in the unit to conduct your reflexive sessions. In the case of the community study (see Vignette 5.3), these moments were sometimes impromptu sessions that took place towards the end of the day when the researcher found some time to edit footage in an open area of the office. This often resulted in a small gathering of clinicians around the laptop discussing the footage while it was being edited. In the study described in Vignette 6.1, researchers together with the clinical team set up a viewing room accessible to the ward to enable video-reflexive sessions to occur together with the medical team immediately after the ward round.

Vignette 6.1 One project, different reflexive session arrangements

Title of project	Strengthening front-line clinicians' infection control: A multi-method study to reduce MRSA infection and transmission (2011–2016)
Researchers	S. Hor, M. Wyer, GL. Gilbert, C. Jorm, C. Hooker, M. O'Sullivan, R. Iedema
	Administering institutions: University of Technology, Sydney, Australia, University of Tasmania, Hobart, Australia
Funder	National Health and Medical Research Council of Australia
Aims of study	To use VRE to increase front-line clinicians' awareness of infection risks and to engage them in designing local improvements to strengthen infection prevention and control
Participants	Clinical and non-clinical staff as well as patients and visitors
Field site	Three different wards at two metropolitan hospitals in Sydney, Australia
Finding suitable space for reflexive sessions	Part of this study involved videoing doctors' surgical rounds on the inpatient unit. These rounds often took place in the early morning and were the only time that the team might be together in one place for the rest of the day. While they were interested in the research, these doctors had a full schedule and little time to view footage. Rather than the researcher taking the footage away and making it into clips before showing these back to the team, she held reflexive sessions with raw footage immediately after the round. This meant finding a suitable space not too far from the ward and having a second researcher available to set that space up ready with computer and projector so that the reflexive session could begin immediately
Publications	Iedema et al. (2018), Iedema et al. (2015), Hor et al. (2017), Gilbert et al. (in preparation)

Another example revealing a different style of reflexive session in the same project occurred during work done in the renal dialysis unit. Here, there was little crossover time between shifts, and nurses were understandably reluctant to leave patients who were connected to dialysis machines and in need of close observation. Staff suggested that 11:00 am was a quiet time in the unit and that if the reflexive sessions could be held at the main nurses' desk, staff could participate in the reflexive activity while also being able to keep an eye on the patients.

A flexible approach to reflexive session arrangements can also be helpful in clinic environments where staff are never sure when patients might arrive. For example, staff in an emergency department asked researchers to assist them by using VRE to help implement a new model of handover. Night to morning shift handovers were videoed, but the doctors and nurses only had around 15 min to view footage and discuss it before their work began in earnest. The research team secured a large empty examination room inside the main emergency department and quickly set up projection of the footage onto a wall. Around 20 staff members were able to attend the session and a productive session was held before the teams dispersed.

You may also need to consider those staff who are not usually available during the day. Will you attend the ward or unit overnight to provide an opportunity for night staff to participate? If you are involving patients and families in reflexive sessions, you will also need to think about 'going to them'. This may be at the bedside, in the clinic or perhaps in the patient's home (see Vignette 6.2).

Vignette 6.2 Going to a patient's home to hold video-reflexive sessions

Title of project	Respect and shared decision-making in the clinical encounter: A video-reflexive ethnographic study
Researchers, Institutions	H. McLeod, University of Minnesota, Minneapolis, Minnesota, USA; Mayo Clinic, Rochester, Minnesota, USA (PhD study)
Aims of study	To describe what respect means to both patients and clinicians and to determine whether respect is related to shared decision-making in primary care clinical encounters
Participants	Patients, caregivers and clinicians
Field site	Primary care clinic in a large academic health system in Minnesota
Going to the patient's residence	• Patient participants were recruited if they consented to having their primary care clinical encounters video-recorded and if they were able to return to a large conference room in

(Continued)

Vignette 6.2 (*Continued*)   Going to a patient's home to hold video-reflexive sessions

the hospital for the video-reflexive sessions. This criterion led to selection bias when patients were unable to return to the hospital setting, for example, if it was a challenge to travel independently. To mitigate this bias, the researcher also met patients in their homes.

- The flexibility of the methodology allowed the researcher to literally 'meet patients where they are' in their homes.
- The size of the room and the screen used to review the edited video-graphic data influenced the reflexive meeting dynamics. In the hospital conference room with an overhead projector, large screen and table separating the researcher and patient, it felt that patients became the object of the research. Whereas in the more familiar setting of a patient's living room, seated together in front of a small laptop, a sense of intimacy was created and the patient appeared to be more of a research collaborator than an object.
- Indeed, as much as setting can influence interaction dynamics, the patient's residence may mitigate the power differential between the researcher and the patient, and transfer some of the initiative to the patient as co-collaborator. Patient participants may feel more comfortable in their home environment and be more open with the researcher.
- Conducting research in the patient's home environment without the highly professionalized audiovisual support of the clinic can present its own research challenges. The researcher will need to work with patients to ensure that the audiovisual technology is appropriate. For example, for older, hearing impaired patients, the audio from the laptop should be adequate, and if necessary, additional speakers may be acquired prior to the home visit

Publications   McLeod (2017)

6.2.1 Reflexive sessions with patients and families

Depending on the context and aim of VRE, there are a variety of ways of engaging patients and families in VRE. In an end-of-life care study (Collier, 2013), patients and families were involved in videoing and sharing of their experiences of care with individual clinicians who were or had been responsible for their care, as well as other groups of clinicians and healthcare workers. Much research now makes use of videoed patient and family narratives of care for motivating practice change (Bate and Robert, 2007; Neuwirth et al., 2012). Collier extended this practice by asking patients to view their own narrative accounts of their care and to become more actively involved in deciding what would be shown back to the clinicians (Collier, 2013). Interestingly, viewing footage turned out to have a transformative effect also on some patients. This happened when they became more aware of their expertise on what constitutes patient-centred care and how this expertise could benefit others, including professionals (Collier and Wyer, 2016).

In the study described in Chapter 5 (Vignette 5.2), patients were invited to analyze the footage of their own clinical care and to look for cross-contamination risks. In this study, the VRE methodology was extended by providing opportunities for clinicians to watch the footage of patients' analyses of their own care, alongside the footage of clinical interactions with patients in group reflexive sessions, thus shrinking the patient/clinician feedback loop. Danielle Bywaters (University of Tasmania, Australia) has been influenced by Wyer's methodological approach through the inclusion of the reflexive session with the patient, and similarly video records herself interacting with the patient whilst watching the original footage of the nurse/patient interaction. In the reflexive session with the nurse, the methodology is applied differently again – rather than in a group forum, the nurse and Bywaters discuss together the original section of the video-recorded interaction between the nurse and a patient, and then the video-recorded patient experience. This reflexive session with the nurse is also video recorded (see Vignette 6.3).

Vignette 6.3   The older person's experience of nurse-led healthcare information sharing

Title of project	The older person's experience of nurse-led healthcare information sharing: A video-reflexive ethnographic study (PhD study 2014–current)
Researchers, Institutions	Danielle Bywaters (PhD candidate), University of Tasmania, Launceston, Australia
	Supervisors: Shandell Elmer, Megan Quentin-Baxter, Aileen Collier
Aims of study	To explore how a video-reflexive methodology can be applied to identify the factors which enable and inhibit learning within an educational encounter, between a specialist nurse and an older person with chronic disease

(Continued)

Vignette 6.3 (*Continued*) The older person's experience of nurse-led healthcare information sharing

Participants	Five specialist nurses and ten patients with chronic disease. Two stomal therapists, one respiratory nurse, one cardiology nurse and one stroke nurse. All of these nurses were involved in semi-structured interviews (audio-recorded). An interaction between a specialist nurse and a patient (65 years of age and over) was video recorded. The stomal therapist with one patient, the cardiology nurse with eight older people with cardiovascular disease and the stroke nurse with one older person with cardiovascular disease. Nine patients participated in the reflexive sessions
Field site	A regional and rural public teaching hospital in Launceston (300 beds), Tasmania, Australia
	Settings: Coronary Care Unit, Stroke Unit, Nurse-led Outpatient Cardiology Clinic, Nurse-led Cancer Surveillance Clinic
Study	The research is designed to determine how the older person understood the healthcare information communicated by the specialist nurse within an educational encounter.
	An educational encounter between a nurse and a patient was video recorded in a clinical setting. Before the researcher showed the video-recorded interaction to the patient, a series of questions were asked, termed the pre-reflexive interview. The purpose was to determine which part of the nurse-led consultation was identified by the patient as most important to the management of their health. Then this section of the video recording was shown to the patient in the first reflexive sessions. Whilst the patient watched the video recording with themself and the nurse, in the interaction the researcher asked probing questions and this discussion which ensued was video recorded
	In the second reflexive session, the nurse watched two video recordings. Firstly, their interaction with the patient, and secondly, the video recording of the patient's responses. The patient's account of the nurse-led consultation is most significant, as this provides the nurse with the opportunity to find out whether the healthcare information which was communicated by them in the initial nurse-led consultation was understood by the patient
Publications	McLeod et al. (2016)

Whether engaging with patients and families during inpatient hospitalization or visiting people in their homes, care must be taken to find a balance between providing opportunities for patients to be involved in research and being respectful of their state of health and treatment plans. A patient's state of health can fluctuate from day to day and sometimes from hour to hour. A patient might commit to a time and place for a reflexive session and then feel too unwell when the time comes. They may be discharged before the reflexive session takes place, or they might simply just change their mind and withdraw from a study.

Likewise, diagnostic tests and treatments are not always planned at fixed times, and the medical team may arrive at unexpected times for their patient rounds. A tension can exist between the researchers respecting patients' and family members' autonomy to decide how involved they want to be in the research and remaining sensitive to the burden that research work can place upon them. Although the aim is for patients to drive the research, it is important to keep checking in with them as to their availability, how well they feel and how they would like to continue be involved in the research. Understanding and respecting patients' rest periods and discussing planned procedures with nursing or medical staff is also important. Box 6.1 shows an example of how a researcher and a patient both negotiated and cancelled a planned reflexive session.

In hospital-based projects, the location for reflexive sessions with patients and families are negotiated with them and are often conducted at the bedside. This is often the most comfortable place for a patient but can present challenges too. Shared rooms can result in tight bed spaces and finding space for laptops and recording equipment can be difficult. Let's consider in greater detail the dynamics of reflexive sessions, before moving on to questions about whether and how to film the reflexive session.

BOX 6.1: Cancelling a reflexive session

A PLANNED SESSION THAT NEEDED TO BE CANCELLED (MARY WYER)

I arrived on the ward to engage in a reflexive session with a patient who had had a procedure videoed a few days before. When I arrived, I found that the patient had undergone surgery earlier than planned. She insisted that she wanted to uphold her commitment to the research and go ahead with the reflexive session, but I could see that she was really unwell. I sat with her and suggested that while the research was important and it was up to her whether she wanted to go ahead – that perhaps it was more important that she concentrated on recovering from surgery at this time. She agreed to cancel our session. Then, she was discharged before we could arrange another time.

6.3 FACILITATING REFLEXIVE SESSIONS

Imagine you have arranged your reflexive session and you have been told that a good number of people are coming. After welcoming everyone and making introductions, you will need to provide people with a detailed sense of what to expect. Give an explanation of what the session is about and provide an overview of what will happen: you are going to show some footage, and they are going to discuss what they see. You might create a PowerPoint presentation or another kind of presentation to structure the session, indicating that you'll focus on some aspects of practice first before moving on to other things. You may want to include a collage of video clips and interview quotes in your slide show. We find it helpful to remind people of the specific project or study, and in particular to remind participants that you have gained consent for both the videoing and the showing of footage. We suggest you make a point of acknowledging the participants who were willing to be videoed and their practices reviewed for the benefit of the team, in what can be a complex and often highly stressful healthcare environment.

Participants usually find it helpful to know what is expected of them during the session. Hence, we often frame the session as a participatory-reflexive exercise to be primarily *led* by participants and facilitated by researcher (and/or another appropriate nominated person). As facilitator, you can emphasize that the session offers a chance to discuss and explore an area of interest to them and could open up the possibility of new ways of looking at care and practices. It is also a space where they as a team can determine a new norm, a new statement of practice or a resolution, in order to 'move on' and mobilize their learning.

To optimize your reflexive session, think about where you will stand or sit during the session and try to create as inclusive an environment as possible. Although you might not have a choice at times, standing behind a lectern as a 'presenter' may not be conducive to the kinds of participatory discussion we aim to generate during reflexive sessions.

Also think about how you might show the clips you have prepared. Stopping a clip in the middle may enable participants to comment on specific facets of the footage. Showing a clip more than once allows participants more time to absorb and reflect on what they see. You may also like to experiment with different approaches, such as watching a clip first with sound and again with sound switched off and encouraging people to talk while watching the soundless clip.

You may also find it helpful to have some prompts ready, for example, questions such as What do you see happening here in this clip? Does anything surprise you? Is there anything the clip should show but does not show? How does watching the clip make you feel?

Overall, we find that the polysemic character of footage will draw people out to enunciate their different views on what is shown. Earlier, we also touched on the hologrammatic affordance of video, enabling people to see pasts, habits, contexts, systems, consequences and futures. All this is likely to enable you to elicit discussion about issues that will go beyond what is seen and heard on the screen.

In Box 6.2, we provide some ideas about the language you can use to kick-start the reflexive discussion. Don't be surprised if you don't get an immediate response from the group, and find that you have to steer the initial conversation. By the same token, do not be afraid of silence. People may still be taking in what they have seen and thinking about it before speaking. Make sure you strike a balance between steering and 'stepping back'. Allow a free flow of discussion as much as possible. Given that people are busy, keeping to the schedule you were allocated is important and always leave time for final questions.

As with any facilitated group situation, you'll need to think about group dynamics and how you will respond if the discussion raises controversies or gets heated. Clinicians can sometimes feel vulnerable when watching themselves. They may feel particularly vulnerable about what patients have to say about aspects of care. In VRE studies that have provided patient feedback to staff, researchers have found it helpful to remind staff that patients have volunteered their time and energy to help us find ways to provide more patient-centred care. Staff were also asked to put on a 'patient hat' (to put themselves in the position of a patient) which helped them to view the feedback as a learning opportunity rather than as criticism. Box 6.2 sets out some helpful guiding questions.

At times, reflexive discussions can seem to lead to too many possibilities, where more and more perspectives lead to more complications, more problems and then still more ideas and strategies. In these situations, discussions can expand to such an extent that participants (and even researchers) feel somewhat weighed down by the complexity they have uncovered. In these situations, it may be helpful to limit the process of reflexive discussion and

---

BOX 6.2: Guiding questions

Example guiding questions

- Can you describe for me what's happening in this clip?
- Is this what usually happens?
- Does anything surprise you in this clip?
- Is there anything that this clip does not show, which is important for understanding what is going on?
- If the person or people videoed is/are present, ask, what were you thinking/feeling when this was happening?
- Ask more research/project-specific questions (which you might distribute beforehand to participants).

awareness expansion. Doing so involves 'contracting' the discussion more towards a consensus about what matters and about what needs to be done. This can be done, for instance, by asking for agreement about what are appropriate strategies to implement or trial, or what could be useful for deciding on next steps for action.

In Table 6.1, we give some examples of language that facilitators can use to moderate reflexive sessions. Drawing on a typology developed by White, the examples include statements that elicit more discussion and ones that tend towards closure (White, 2003). White refers to 'dialogic' utterances (statements that encourage discussion) and 'monologic' utterances (statements that close a conversation down). Dialogic statements are useful for taking stock and for ensuring that the group agrees on what has been said. Dialogic statements are also useful for encouraging participants to expand their comments and continue their line of thinking.

Statements which act to 'close' the discussion by not accepting additional perspectives or ideas can be useful, for instance, when you need to put a stop to the discussion because you're running out of time, or because you need to draw a boundary around the discussion to maintain a safe space for participants.

It is important to remember that facilitating reflexive sessions can be unnerving. Participants may have fixed ideas about aspects of their work, and reflecting on these may not be easy for them. For this reason, it is important to reflect on specific participants' vulnerabilities to make sure that you know what to look out for as and when your session unfolds. Box 6.3 sets out some questions to help you think about this.

Table 6.1 Moderating language for reflexive session facilitators

Statement type	Function	Examples
Dialogic (opening up) statements	'taking stock'	• (Summarizing statements such as) 'So in other words', 'Do you mean...' • 'What do you think was your/their priority in this situation?'
	'expanding'	• 'How do you feel about that [shown on the screen], is that something you might ordinarily do or see?' • 'Does anyone do/see things differently?' • 'What might patients/visitors/other staff think of that?' • 'What could we do about this, you personally or your team?'
Monologic statements	'closing down'	• 'Okay. Let's move on'. • 'In the interest of time, let's wrap up'. • 'This session is not about blaming individuals for their mistakes'.

> **BOX 6.3: Questions to consider when dealing with people's vulnerabilities**
>
> - How might your collaborators be vulnerable to discomfort during this project? (e.g. was their videoed behaviour criticized (by them or by others)? were their suggestions not responded to or not taken seriously?)
> - How might you and your project team be vulnerable to discomfort during this project? (e.g. participants may challenge your choice of clips or your explanations about them)
> - What other risks of harm might there be to people taking part in the project? (e.g. idiosyncratic behaviours may now be public)
> - Are there risks of harm to people who do not want to participate? (e.g. the stigma of non-participation)
> - How can you create 'psychological safety' (Edmondson, 1999) at every stage of the project for your collaborators?
> - How vulnerable are junior staff, staff who may feel powerless (e.g. cleaners) and patients and visitors who are dependent on hospital care?

6.4 REFLEXIVITY COMPETENCIES

Reflexive sessions may spark people into participating in ways they themselves might not have thought possible. The sessions may inspire interest, enthusiasm, even laughter, upon people seeing themselves and realizing there is a whole world out there of behaviours, habits, practices and systems that they have been taking for granted. In our experience, this revelation often leads to people beginning to enjoy seeing themselves and each other, and they may forget about time constraints and spend the next several hours discussing what you've shown them. Several days if not weeks later, you may run into them and hear them talking about what you've shown them and the discussion you elicited from them.

In our 2013 book, we cited the following description from a 1999 paper by Innes and Booher (1999) on consensus building. The description captures the kind of creative dynamic that we may witness during reflexive sessions. Innes and Booher describe the consensus building dynamic that is their focus of interest using the French word *bricolage*, which means something like tinkering, cobbling together. We cite the passage again here, to pick up in what follows on some of the behaviours that may enable and support bricolage.

> In their most productive moments, participants in consensus building engage not only in playing out scenarios, but also in a kind of collective, speculative tinkering, or bricolage ... That is, they play with heterogeneous concepts, strategies and actions with which various individuals in the group have experience, and try combining them until they create a new scenario that they collectively believe will work. This bricolage ... is a type of reasoning and collective

creativity fundamentally different from the more familiar types, argumentation and trade-offs ... Bricolage ... produces, rather than a solution to a known problem, a new way of framing the situation and of developing unanticipated combinations of actions that are qualitatively different from the options on the table at the outset. The result ... is, most importantly, learning and change among the players, and growth in their sophistication about each other, about the issues, and about the futures they could seek.

(Innes and Booher, 1999: 12)

The connection between consensus building and reflexive discussion can be construed as follows: For the former (consensus building), a creative, innovative process called bricolage is the condition for the group producing a novel consensus agreement. (While expertly describing the dynamics of that process, the passage above leaves undisclosed ways in which we can enable people to become creative and innovative.) In contrast, the latter (the VRE reflexive session) provides evidence of 'what is' (video footage), encouraging and enabling people to re-apprehend and more deeply appreciate 'what is'. This, as explained, asks them to 'exnovate': to pay attention to the aspects of existing practice and behaviour that have been taken for granted. This engagement with 'what is', we suggest, is the condition par excellence for eliciting exnovation, that is, for new insight, creativity and, ultimately, consensus to become possible 'about the futures they could seek' (Innes and Booher, 1999: 12).

Let us try to unpack this bricolage, or 'speculative tinkering,' still further so that we can specify what reflexivity looks like as *in situ* dynamic. In doing so, we can try to frame the kind of discussion we'd hope to see taking place in relation to a set of requisite competences or conditions, if you like. Table 6.2 sets out a list of such competences and conditions. The question marks indicate the possibility that the relevant competence applies not just to facilitators but also to participants. Note that some competences and conditions are structural (e.g. 'timing'), others are discursive (e.g. 'reframing what is said', 'resemiotizing agreements

Table 6.2 Conditions for reflexive sessions to realize exnovation

Strategies/tactics	Facilitator behaviour	Participant behaviour
Taking time to ascertain the representativeness of the footage shown	√	
Framing responses to the footage in non-categorical ways	√	√
Active listening by giving others' time to express ideas, concerns, positions, interests, etc.	√	√

(Continued)

Table 6.2 (*Continued*) Conditions for reflexive sessions to realize exnovation

Strategies/tactics	Facilitator behaviour	Participant behaviour
Responding nonjudgmentally to participants' novel ideas and insights	√	√
Checking through summarizing what has been said	√	
Reframing what has been said to open up new vistas for thought and action	√	
Remaining attuned constantly to the affective dynamics driving the discussion	√	?
Capitalizing on enthusiasm realized as intensified participation while	√	
Monitoring and mitigating excessive assertiveness and insufficient mutual responsiveness and questioning	√	?
Heading off tension through alternating yielding, questioning and claiming/stating	√	?
Modulating others' contributions ensuring the discussion alternates yielding, questioning and claiming/stating	√	
Recognizing and using questions posed to others as entry points into openness	√	√
Collecting and confirming agreements through 'resemiotizing' them, that is, recasting them from verbal to written to diagrammatic forms	√	?
Timing the discussion and structuring it accordingly by changing gears from total openness, to engaged openness, to inchoate closing off, to emergent closure	√	
Outlining strategies for revisiting issues and follow-up	√	?

from talk into writing'), whereas again others are emotional or affective (e.g. 'responding nonjudgmentally', 'heading off tension').

While we would expect facilitators and participants to adjust their behaviour to realize these competences to satisfy the necessary conditions, some competences may be more typical of what facilitators (should) do (e.g. summarizing, reframing, capitalizing on enthusiasm, monitoring excessive assertiveness, heading off tensions, timing, and so on), and others may be more typical of what participants (should) do (e.g. responding to footage in nonjudgmental ways, active listening, and so forth). Understandably, in projects that aim for obsolescence, the necessary task for facilitators is to transfer these competences to co-researchers and participants.

6.5 CAPTURING THE REFLEXIVE SESSION ON VIDEO

Having provided an outline of what a productive reflexive session sounds and feels like, we now move on to the issue of recording the reflexive session. Videoed reflexive sessions may be regarded as a record of you and your participants responding to and co-analyzing footage, and negotiating responses and insights. Videoing the reflexive session enables the research team to look back, summarize and analyze further what happened and work out how to assist with possible future action. It also enables facilitators to reflect on their own performance (see Section 6.6). For this reason and with permission of participants, these sessions are often videoed. It is important to explain why you are doing so however. Participant consent to videoing reflexive sessions requires formal as well as situational realization of ethical practice. Even if some participants present have already consented formally as part of the videoing phase, you need to check with them again verbally that they consent to being videoed again.

Of course, if people are not comfortable with being videoed during the session, you can audio record instead. If there are some people who are happy to be videoed and others not, you can ask those who would prefer not to be videoed to sit out of camera range. If there are participants attending who have not yet provided consent, you will need to gain their written consent, so it's always a good idea to bring some information sheets and consent forms to the session itself, and allocate time to explaining and completing the paperwork.

While one of the main goals of the session is to understand the participants' perspectives on the footage, if you are videoing the reflexive session, you will also need to think ahead to how this footage will look like to anyone else you might present it to – be that to clinicians during reflexive sessions, at conferences or in publications. Some researchers position themselves on camera with the participant to emphasize, to subsequent viewers, the co-analysis by researcher and participant of the video footage (Collier and Wyer, 2016). Consider also whether your camera is able to capture, in the close range of a confined space, the people involved in the reflexive session as well as the laptop you are viewing. The resulting footage will make it easier for subsequent viewers to understand the event.

Dilemmas may arise however in the spaces where you conduct your reflexive session. Earlier, we considered dilemmas encountered when capturing reflexive discussions with staff in hospital and primary care spaces. Dilemmas may arise in other spaces too. Figures 6.1 and 6.2 show examples of very different results obtained when capturing reflexive sessions with patients. Figure 6.1 shows that in this instance the camera was well placed to capture the proceedings in a patient's home. In contrast, Figure 6.2 shows a situation, in a patient's private room, where a laptop that is not part of the reflexive session occupies a central position on the screen. To avoid problems like the one encountered here, always consider where you place the camera and how useful the resulting footage will be for you afterwards.

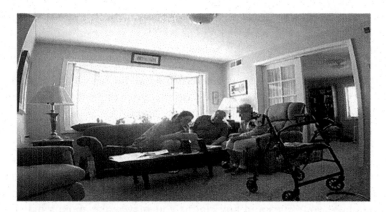

Figure 6.1 Example of an effectively captured reflexive session – Patients reviewing footage with researcher in a patient's home. (Picture courtesy of Heidi McLeod, Geisinger Health System, Danville, Pennsylvania, USA.)

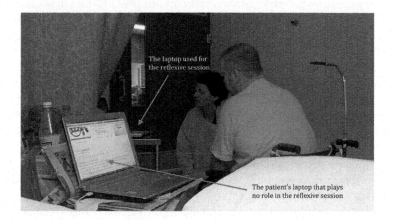

Figure 6.2 Example of an ineffectively captured reflexive session – The laptop that the researcher and patient are viewing is hidden behind the patient's own laptop which is in the foreground. This often confuses people watching this footage. (Picture courtesy of Mary Wyer.)

Privacy can also be an issue, particularly when people are about to engage in discussions that enable them to say and think new things. When involving clinicians, always make sure your space has adequate privacy. When involving patients and families, consider their privacy particularly when curtains are sometimes the only divider between you and the other patients in the room and the staff that are working there.

Discuss with participants how comfortable they feel in the chosen environment, how free they feel to discuss what they see in the footage and how comfortable they are being videoed. It may be possible to find another quiet room to do the session or arrange to meet in another location. If you are conducting reflexive sessions in a patient's private room, there will be more space and privacy. However, if the patient is in a single room on infection transmission precautions, be mindful of the facility's infection prevention and control standards, particularly in relation to the equipment that you want to use.

Finally, if you are unable to video-record or audio-record the session think about how you will keep track of the discussion, and of people's ideas for improvement. You may need to enlist someone to take notes.

6.6 RESEARCHER AND PARTICIPANT REFLEXIVITY

As noted in Section 4.9, as a researcher or practice improvement clinician, you make yourself vulnerable through your choice of clips, your explanation about how you chose your clips and any claims you may make about what the clips represent (Carroll, 2009a; Carroll, 2009b). Where common kinds of research and improvement tend to limit people's and especially researchers' vulnerability, VRE maximizes people's vulnerability. Conventional approaches tend to persuade people by presenting (often large amounts of) formal data, discipline-specific analyses and supportable conclusions. These approaches do not often prioritize creative discussion and bricolage.

As described in Chapter 4, the process of producing video clips and the way in which we present them to audiences are, inevitably, processes of analysis and reflect our (and ideally our participants') decisions. Recognizing that footage is invariably constructed (even in its 'raw' state) means that the relevance, representativeness and meaning of your footage may be questioned, even rejected by participants. Inevitably, your clip choices and presentation will be closely watched by your audience and especially by those whom you have chosen to represent in your footage. Keep in mind though that their critical responses may reflect their own sense of discomfort resulting from being confronted with watching themselves and engaging in reflexivity – activities that may be alien to them and counter to their self-identity and professional status. This is why collaboration at every step of the way is critical, as is managing the emotional dynamics of the reflexive session. It is also important for you to reflect on your own behaviour, reactions and responses.

> Reflexivity is paying attention to every step of the research process, particularly to the fact that you yourself are doing it (whether you are asking questions or identifying a code or building an argument or crafting a sentence) and then making an account of what you actually did ... Reflexivity is taking responsibility for your research.
>
> *(Carter, 2010: 147)*

Carter's quote suggests that engendering questioning attitudes should apply as much to researchers as it does to participants. VRE presents a special case in this regard. The VRE process is never straightforward: as much as you can plan ahead and gather information, you never know what is actually going to happen when you go into complex healthcare settings and try to intervene in them. To put it in a nutshell, the very requirement of researcher–participant entanglement means that VRE will be complex and messy. This means, in effect, that every 'in the moment' decision and/or response that you as facilitator make, can also give rise to questions and, in turn, produce new dilemmas.

For example, consider again Vignette 5.3, where the researchers involved the palliative care team in a reflexivity session in an already existing education slot. This meeting, which had been in place for some time, had existing normative social dynamics including power differentials between and within different disciplines in the team. This had implications for who got to have a say and whose say mattered. It was important for the researcher to reflect on these dynamics and on how their behaviours normalized or reconfigured these dynamics.

Holding the reflexive session in an already existing meeting also has implications for how to obtain consent. For example, is it possible, particularly on a first occasion, that all staff are adequately prepared for such session? Might they walk into the room and realize the atmosphere effectively prevents them from speaking freely? Will staff feel able to withdraw from the session? Indeed, what does being fully 'prepared' for a session mean, and how should a facilitator go about consenting people for a group video-reflexive session? Box 6.4 offers some key questions in this regard that you can ask yourself to reflect on how your reflexive session could or did unfold.

BOX 6.4: Questions for the reflexive researcher

- How do/did the decisions about meeting arrangements impact on participants' ability to speak freely?
- How do/did the decisions I/we made about clips/editing/timing, etc. affect the reflexive session?
- How do/did I/we represent people in the clips?
- How do/might participants feel about the session?
- Should I show/have shown a particular clip to a particular audience even though I have consent from the person in it?
- How much of a say will/did participants have and will/did they all have opportunities to participate?
- What will/did I learn from participating in the reflexive session? Have I been transformed in any way by participating in the session and if so how?
- When I watch back the footage of reflexive sessions, how is my facilitation? Have I tried to fill silences and put words in people's mouths? How has that influenced the session and does it matter and to who?
- What are the relationships that have or could have developed as a result of the session?

6.7 WHEN THINGS DON'T GO AS PLANNED

Things don't always go quite to plan. Perhaps no one turns up to the reflexive session, or you have waited patiently for days for an appropriate time to have a session with a patient, and they are discharged from hospital before you get the chance to speak with them. Or worse, you have spent weeks preparing the site, and out of the blue, a senior clinician returns from leave and refuses to let the team participate. Here, in this section, we share some of our less favourable experiences and what we have learned from them.

EXAMPLE 1 – INTERRUPTIONS AND THE INTENSIVE CARE UNIT (SU-YIN HOR)

I had organized a reflexive session to be intentionally interdisciplinary and to include the nurse unit manager, two junior doctors and several ward nurses with the aim of looking at footage concerning interruptions. A group of nursing students who were asked to attend as part of their learning were also present. Ironically, just as the session began, an alarm went off and both junior doctors and the nurse manager left the room, rightly so, but never returned. This left me as a researcher with six nursing students who didn't speak, a ward nurse who was new to the project and reluctant to talk and one very enthusiastic nurse who had a great deal to say and who had a lovely time expounding on his reflections on the footage.

KEY LEARNING

Despite being not at what I had planned and hoped for, I'm reluctant to consider this session a failure. Rather, it exemplified the nature of clinical practice in this ward. The problem (interruptions) ended up being of great interest in subsequent (more successful) multidisciplinary reflexive sessions. I reflected on this experience and organized and publicized subsequent sessions more broadly and widely ahead of time – to ensure that more people were able to attend, allowing for a representative group, even if some were called away during the meetings.

EXAMPLE 2 – THE ACUTE HOSPITAL – CONFLICT AND THE RESEARCHER AGENDA (KATHERINE CARROLL, THEN A RECENTLY RETIRED PHYSIOTHERAPIST)

During my PhD project, I noticed how the allied health professionals operated at the periphery of intensive care. This bothered me, and it bothered the allied health as 'we' knew that if we had earlier access to this intensive care unit (ICU) patient population, we could enhance their outcomes and speed up their hospital discharge. However, delayed discharge did not seem to bother the medical specialists. I had 'amazing' data from allied health on what they *could do* for these patients should they be more incorporated culturally and financially into the unit's processes and practices. However, the medical specialists were in control of those processes and practices. So I set myself up as a cultural broker between the allied health staff and the specialists. I used a VRE session to show what allied health could do for ICU patients. I had terrific data, and good intentions, but allied health intervention was not deemed a priority by the single specialist who chose to attend my session. In fact, the specialist responded angrily to my presentation and accused me of beating the 'medical dominance' drum. This outburst silenced all the other attending staff and me.

KEY LEARNING

At the conclusion of the reflexive session, other attendees came up to me to inform me that the specialist was really not a fan of allied health in the unit and that his view was not shared by other specialists. It was just bad luck that I had this one person attend, and that he was the most senior clinician in the room at the time. The next day, the specialist did come and apologize to me for his outburst and try and make things right. But the VRE session was forever ruined. I acknowledge that I had unwittingly brought up a sensitive issue, but I had hoped it might have resulted in practice change. I think I let my identity as a recently retired physiotherapist interfere with my approach to the reflexive session. Ever since, I have been very consultative in my approach to all aspects of VRE.

EXAMPLE 3 – PATIENTS, FAMILIES AND CLINICIANS – POWER DIFFERENTIALS (AILEEN COLLIER)

As part of my PhD, I recruited a patient and spouse who I had collaborated with me over some months. A clinical team contributing to this person's care invited me to give a presentation of the research in their workplace. With their permission, I included the footage of the couple's experiences of the service, which were extremely positive. My view was that if I was to show back the couple's footage along with some broader findings in this meeting, then it was only 'right' to invite them along. They would be the only service users at the meeting and I gave the invitation careful consideration. On balance however, I decided to invite them, explain to them who would be there and let them decide whether to accept my invitation or not. Given the power differential in the room, and in the knowledge the couple might not feel able to speak up, I offered them the first opportunity to respond to footage. I was unprepared for what happened next. The patient not only felt able to speak up; they strongly expressed their feelings about the closure of one particular component of the service. They clearly articulated what this component of the service had meant to them. At that moment, I felt impressed that this participant had been able to speak up about how she felt despite being in a room full of clinicians. The clinicians, on the other hand, were extremely upset. They were obviously uncomfortable and felt I had put them in a very difficult situation and they had little control over that situation. The director of the service communicated to me by email that the incident had been a difficult one that could have caused significant damage.

KEY LEARNING

At the time I felt I had completely damaged the relationship with the service provider. As difficult as it was, I made a time to meet the service medical director to apologize for placing her and her medical colleagues in a difficult situation. We were able to have an honest and productive discussion. This was to become a pivotal moment in our relationship – we continue to collaborate as research peers today! Would or could I have done anything differently to prevent this from happening? Perhaps I could have been clearer in my communication to the facilitator of the meeting and/or the service director that I had invited the couple and what footage contained. I was unaware of the service changes, and perhaps the director of the service would have been able to inform me about these changes had I communicated my plans more clearly. Yet this is all with the benefit of hindsight. Nonetheless and on reflection, I'm not sure the research participants had an issue in this scenario. Looking at it from their perspective, the session allowed them to publicly convey their opinions, thoughts and feelings about the changes. I'm not so sure that was a bad thing. I wonder whether this was simply about clinicians' vulnerability and unease about articulating and negotiating emotion.

6.8 FINAL FEEDBACK SESSIONS TO CLOSE YOUR PROJECT

Some VRE projects include one or more final close-of-project 'feedback' reflexive sessions. These final sessions draw from the combined findings of the project observations, interviews and reflexive sessions to present to participants the main potentials, challenges and solutions that have been identified. These sessions can be especially useful for bringing common themes, problems and solutions to the attention of managers, who can or should be able to sanction and action change, if they have not been overly involved in the project up to this point. These sessions can also be a way of showcasing to them the creativity and expertise of ward staff and patients for creating and maintaining safety as well as a way of accounting for the research activities to date.

6.9 CONCLUSION

This chapter has detailed the issues that arise when you conduct your reflexive sessions. The chapter has set out some practical advice, and it has discussed the kinds of competences and conditions that have to be realized for the reflexive discussion to unfold in ways that are authentic, sensitive and productive. The chapter has further described cases where reflexive sessions were less than successful. Chapter 7 moves on to considering the issues that arise when we want to evaluate VRE projects, and it lists some notable VRE achievements.

REFERENCES

Bate P and Robert G. (2007) *Bringing User Experience to Healthcare Improvement: The Concepts, Methods and Practices of Experience-Based Design*. Oxford/Seattle, WA: Radcliffe.

Carroll K. (2009a) Outsider, insider, alongsider: Examining reflexivity in hospital-based video research. *International Journal of Multiple Research Approaches* 3: 246–263.

Carroll K. (2009b) Unpredictable predictables: Complexity theory and the construction of order in intensive care. Unpublished PhD Thesis. Sydney: Centre for Health Communication, University of Technology Sydney.

Carter S. (2010) Enacting internal coherence as a path to quality in qualitative inquiry. In: Higgs J, Cherry C, Macklin R, et al. (eds) *Researching Practice: A Discourse on Qualitative Methodologies*. Rotterdam: Sense, 143–152.

Collier A. (2013) Deleuzians of patient safety: A video reflexive ethnography of end-of-life care. PhD Thesis. Sydney: Faculty of Arts and Social Sciences, University of Technology, Sydney.

Collier A and Wyer M. (2016) Researching reflexively with patients and families: Two studies using video-reflexive ethnography to collaborate with patients and families in patient safety research. *Qualitative Health Research* 26: 979–993.

Edmondson A. (1999) Psychological safety and learning behavior in work teams. *Administrative Science Quarterly* 44(2): 350–383.

Gilbert L, O'Sullivan M, Dempsey K, et al. (in preparation) Whatever it takes: A prospective intervention study, using video-reflexive methods (VRM) and enhanced conventional infection prevention and control, to reduce MRSA transmission in two surgical wards.

Hor S, Hooker C, Iedema R, et al. (2017) Beyond hand hygiene: A qualitative study of the everyday work of preventing cross-contamination on hospital wards. *BMJ Quality & Safety* 26: 552–558.

Iedema R, Hor S, Wyer M, et al. (2015) An innovative approach to strengthening health professionals' infection control and limiting hospital acquired infection: Video-reflexive ethnography. *BMJ Innovation*. doi:10.1136/bmjinnov-2014-000032.

Iedema R, Jorm C, Hooker C, et al. (2018). To follow a rule? On frontline clinicians' understandings and embodiments of hospital-acquired infection preventionand control rules. *Health*. doi:10.1177/1363459318785677.

Innes JE and Booher DE. (1999) Consensus building as role playing and bricolage – Toward a collaborative theory of planning. *Journal of the American Planning Association* 65: 9–25.

McLeod H. (2017) Respect and shared decision making in the clinical encounter: A video-reflexive ethnography. PhD Thesis. University of Minnesota.

McLeod H, Bywaters D, Collier A, et al. (2016) The patient revolution and video-reflexive ethnography. In: *ACSPRI Social Science Methodology Conference*. Univerity of Sydney, 19–22 July.

Neuwirth EB, Bellows J, Jackson AH, et al. (2012) How Kaiser Permanente uses video ethnography of patients for quality improvement. *Health Affairs* 31: 1244–1250.

White PRR. (2003) Beyond modality and hedging: A dialogic view of the language of intersubjective stance. *Text* 23: 259–284.

7

Evaluating VRE achievements

7.1 INTRODUCTION

This chapter sets out how to evaluate practical video-reflexive ethnography (VRE) project achievements. This involves first articulating different evaluation approaches and perspectives, and then describing the evaluation models that are most suitable for measuring VRE impact. This section makes clear that VRE projects are difficult to evaluate using conventional metrics. It suggests that, given VRE operates with and amidst maximum complexity, unconventional approaches to evaluation are called for. Section 7.2 summarizes a range of VRE projects' practical outcomes. Here, we briefly summarize the previously published work where these achievements are described in greater detail.

7.2 EVALUATING COMPLEX PROJECTS

The evaluation of the effectiveness of projects that seek to intervene in how healthcare is structured and enacted is challenging. This is because, first, health care is complex in itself. The term 'complex' describes situations where we see a confluence of factors, a lack of clear causation, and a range of emergent (unpredictable) outcomes. Healthcare interventions will somehow have to engage with complexity because patients are becoming more complex (more co-morbidities, more uncertainty), treatments are becoming more complex (think of polypharmacy and intricate kinds of surgery) and care trajectories are becoming more complex (due to more and changing technologies, treatment options, regulations, staff and care sites). Our evaluation of attempts to intervene in this complexity can be based either on the assumption that it is appropriate and necessary to excise complexity from its remit, or on the view that we need to allow complexity to impinge on the unfolding of initiatives and thus account for complexity in our evaluation. These decisions affect our understandings of and conclusions about whether and how an initiative has been worthwhile.

By way of illustration of the point we are making here, consider the introduction of checklists as a solution to reduce surgical incidents. Notwithstanding the complexity of the settings and practices into which checklists were introduced, the uptake of checklists was claimed to lead to a radical reduction in incidents

(Gawande, 2011). At the time, Gawande's *Checklist Manifesto* was hailed as a groundbreaking advance in patient safety. Others, however, have argued that the impact and success of checklists were not at all ensured and straightforward, and that checklists are not as easy an intervention to evaluate as they might appear. This point has been made particularly forcefully by Bosk and colleagues: '[t]he mistake of the "simple checklist" story is in the assumption that a technical solution (checklists) can solve an adaptive (sociocultural) problem' (Bosk et al., 2009: 444). For Bosk and colleagues, evaluating technical solutions relies on very different assumptions and approaches compared to evaluating adaptive sociocultural interventions, of which VRE is one approach.

Sociocultural interventions confront uncertainty in so far as that social actors may not respond in predictable ways, they may change the way they respond to initiatives midway, and their responses may be ambiguous (i.e. uncertain) or even ambivalent (i.e. contradictory). For these reasons, sociocultural initiatives need to take account of local actors' reasoning, assumptions, preferences, intentions, changes of heart and mind and politics. Sociocultural initiatives produce outcomes that may not be conclusive or lasting; their conclusions may not suit particular stakeholders and remain contested and their interpretation may vary among actors and inspire different kinds and levels of uptake.

Put simply, social studies and interventions may harbour considerable complexity and uncertainty. Their evaluation will necessarily also be complex as it will be based not on elegant conclusions and evidence-based outcomes but on more or less careful weighing up of interpretations, experiences and arguments (Mertens, 2009).

The complexity of sociocultural interventions becomes further evident if we think that as soon as we enter the domain of health care, we are likely to encounter a plethora of parallel care activities and priorities that intersect with the one(s) in which we are interested. Health care encompasses multiple professionals and non-health professional stakeholders; there may be an organizational restructuring, and there may be divergent perspectives on what is good in care, on what should stay the way it is and on what warrants changing. Because the study of and intervention in healthcare practice are likely to encounter this type of complexity, and assuming it is unlikely that complexity can be fully excised from their remit, those involved in healthcare research and improvement cannot but take account of *in situ* circumstances and events that impact on and perturb their initiatives. Not surprisingly, there is now growing acknowledgement that context (i.e. the entire ecology of situations, events and circumstances encountered) plays a critical role in how initiatives unfold in real time (Ovretveit, 2011).

To support us in thinking through these issues, the Medical Research Council (MRC) in the United Kingdom published a series of reports offering guidance for designing and evaluating complex interventions (Medical Research Council (UK), 2006). The MRC's general message is as follows: Complex interventions require "a good theoretical understanding" of how the intervention is assumed to cause change, an acknowledgement that failure to register impact may be due to implementation obstacles (such as 'teething problems') and local constraints, rather than inappropriate solution design, among other things. The kinds of

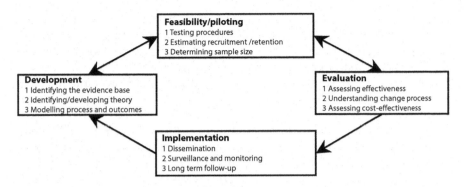

Figure 7.1 MRC's (2006) circular approach to developing, piloting, evaluating and implementing complex interventions. (Reproduced with permission from the Medical Research Council.)

problems that typically associate with complex interventions, the MRC states, include 'the difficulty of standardizing the design and delivery of the interventions, their sensitivity to features of the local context, the organizational and logistical difficulty of applying experimental methods to service or policy change, and the length and complexity of the causal chains linking intervention with outcome' (Medical Research Council (UK), 2006: 6). Figure 7.1, from the 2006 MRC report, sets out this rather linear – if circular – approach to initiative development and evaluation.

Even if we accept the MRC's advice and qualifications, there are numerous difficulties associated with conducting initiatives amidst complex circumstances and carry them out as suggested in Figure 7.1. We may not be sure what has caused improved outcomes or what has prevented outcomes from improving. This uncertainty raises issues for how to evaluate such initiatives and translate their local unfolding into more general learnings.

One way in which this dilemma has been resolved is by qualifying the outcomes with reference to local, contextual influences and constraints. That is, the evaluation of initiatives' outcomes seems to require 'realistic' explanations about why certain outcomes transpired and what local factors might have shaped these outcomes (Pawson and Tilley, 1997).

The term 'realistic' here refers to a stance that acknowledges that no initiative is likely to unfold mechanistically and impervious to real-world circumstances, constraints and perturbations. Pawson and Tilley's 'realistic evaluation' approach was articulated as a way of going beyond the expectations of those who wanted a simple yes/no answer to questions: is this the right thing to do? and does it actually work? Realistic evaluation thus aims to pay due attention to why specific findings or outcomes may have come about, given what is known about the context, circumstances, local events, players and constraints.

A related evaluation approach includes REAIM, an acronym that stands for 'reach, effectiveness, adoption, implementation, and maintenance'. In the literature, the dimensions of REAIM are described as follows: 'the "reach" dimension of the framework refers to the percentage and characteristics of individuals receiving the intervention; "effectiveness" refers to the impact of the intervention, including anticipated as well as unanticipated outcomes; "adoption" concerns the percentage and representativeness of settings that adopt the intervention; "implementation" refers to the consistency and cost of delivering the intervention; and "maintenance" refers to long-term sustainability at both the setting and individual levels' (King et al., 2010: 2076).

Like Pawson and Tilley's realistic evaluation, REAIM operates on the principle that a pre-defined mechanism needs to be evaluated in terms of its impact on a pre-existing real-world state of affairs. That is, for both realistic evaluation and REAIM, the mechanism, the change that is aspired to, is pre-defined, and its legitimacy or effectiveness is determined by scrutinizing its impact on practice processes or on practice outcomes in specific contexts. In essence, this means that the mechanism (the logic underpinning the initiative) is known, singular, uncontested and able to be fully articulated in advance of the study. Equally, the mechanism remains under the control of the team who initiates the project – even though that team may include front-line clinicians, patients and family members. Put bluntly, the mechanism remains more or less predetermined, and its design answers to the assumptions and reasoning of those initiating the project.

7.3 TRANSFORMATIVE RESEARCH AND EVALUATION: *NOTHING ABOUT US WITHOUT US*

We suggest that the approaches just reviewed do not exhaust all possibilities for pursuing and evaluating healthcare initiatives. Alternatives abound. In the first instance, the 'distance' or separation between those who design projects and those who are its recipients or participants can be significantly compressed. One example is provided in the book *Transformative Research and Evaluation* by Donna Mertens (2009). In this book, Mertens sets out a very different way of thinking about how to study and intervene in existing practices and social systems. Mertens' paradigm holds that those who are at the centre of interest for those keen to initiate transformations – say, the clinicians, patients and family members who are party to a particular care practice – should also be central to how the initiative is formulated, conducted and concluded (Mertens, 2009). With this, Mertens espouses the 'nothing about us without us' principle that defines indigenous ethics and research (Chatterji, 2001).

Second, Mertens' paradigm assumes that such initiatives' unfolding is inevitably dynamic and non-linear, given the complexity of stakeholder relationships, social practices and cultural differences. This means that a single intervention design (a single 'mechanism') may not be sufficient. The mechanism may need to be adapted, perhaps even rewritten. Third, stakeholders' involvement is not just informative but *transformative*. Here, it is not simply about participants who provide information and experts who adduce knowledge. Instead, all those involved in the initiative are enabled to express, absorb, change *and evaluate* perspectives, practices and outcomes. In sum, these initiatives' sensitivity and receptiveness to stakeholders' concerns and tensions convert into a dynamic emergence of methods, a co-construction of understandings and interpretations, an iterative negotiation of change mechanisms and project decisions and a co-created evaluation of progress and impact.

As noted, Mertens' paradigm aligns with the indigenous research paradigm whose essence is 'nothing about us without us' (Chatterji, 2001). To connect this principle to VRE, and to add to our discussion in Chapter 2, we confirm that the ethics that governs VRE projects is not an abstract concern that is satisfied once consent forms have been signed. Instead, indigenous research ethics informs VRE in its entirety. Thus, VRE operates on the principle 'nothing about us without us' in terms of how it relates to participants, and this principle governs all of the following: how VRE grants roles to and invites views from participants, how VRE navigates among participants' interests and concerns, what VRE draws on as data, how VRE seeks participants' interpretations and views, how VRE enables participants' learning and how VRE seeks participants' views on VRE initiatives' meaning and impact.

VRE's co-creative approach therefore identifies closely with Mertens' paradigm promoting transformative research and evaluation. VRE pulls back a little, however, from the linguistically and narratively negotiated agreements and understandings that predominate in Mertens' paradigm. Harnessing visualization, VRE operates through observation, the camera, footage and the shared review of *in situ* practice to make possible new perspectives on 'what is' and on 'what may be'. For VRE, the visual medium anchors us to (a version of) 'what is' or 'what was'. This renders VRE somewhat less dependent on people's memories, opinions or narratives than are other approaches, such as Mertens' transformative research and evaluation.

This is also what distinguishes VRE from co-design (Bate and Robert, 2007). Co-design may involve footage of interviews about care experiences that are shown to clinicians and other stakeholders. Essentially, co-design visualizes talk, interviews and narratives about care, rather than visualizing care as it happens. VRE is therefore unique in how it puts the moment-to-moment unfolding of care centre stage and how it makes its intervention dynamics fully contingent on how practitioners and patients respond to the footage and how their realizations and responses then impact on existing identities, practices and systems.

It is important to acknowledge, then, that when it comes to evaluating VRE initiatives, we are not able to evaluate a predetermined intervention and a predefined change. Instead, we have to account for unpredictable effects produced through confronting local actors with existing behaviours, interests, concerns and practices. These effects may include practical improvements, and they may include people's personal realizations (which may not as yet have practical effect), or even psychological transformations that can only be identified through careful elicitation and in-depth narration. These effects may also include significant changes to local practice (Carroll et al., 2008) or interventions whose relevance and uptake extends beyond the original site(s).

Given this potential multiplicity and diversity of effects, measurement of VRE impact is challenging. Measurement presumes the existence and validity of a pre-existing yardstick and a uniformity or at least comparability of impact. Yet uniformity and comparability apply only to pre-designed interventions, rigidly executed plans and narrowly delineated outcomes. Measurement is less suited to ascertain the impact of sociocultural interventions such as VRE facing complex circumstances and engaging with unpredictable developments.

7.4 EVALUATING VRE INITIATIVES

So how might we ascertain the impact of VRE? We noted that, aside from the possibility that VRE produces no change at all, it may occasion change that manifests as emerging awareness of clinicians' personal roles in care practice, psychological change affecting clinicians' identity as professionals, practical alteration of clinicians' ways of working, technological resourcing of spatial context or, indeed, critical structural and systemic changes. Each of these kinds of impacts is described in Section 7.5. Each necessitates a different approach to evaluation.

Where the more personal and interactive effects of VRE on individuals may only become apparent through interviewing or surveying (Iedema et al., 2009), effects on practice may be ascertained through comparative ethnographic observation of team interactive dynamics and communication (Carroll et al., 2008), medical chart and patient trajectory analyses (Neuwirth et al., 2012), studies of cross-infection rates (Gilbert et al., in preparation), reported changes in the conduct and structure of clinical practices (Hor et al., 2014; Wyer et al., 2017) and so forth. Reverberations of effects beyond the participants and the site may become apparent from take-up elsewhere following publications and conference presentations (Gordon et al., 2016) or from new regulatory state-wide standards based on VRE outcomes (Iedema et al., 2012), and the like.

These different evaluation paradigms all have a unique affordance and validity.

With this, we acknowledge that the time has now come for funders, policy makers and academics to become more accepting of variety in how we expedite and evaluate change (Mitchell, 2009). As Greenhalgh and colleagues note: 'a "logic model" mind-set with inflexible goals will be less effective than an approach that acknowledges nonlinearity and encourages local adaptation as the programme unfolds' (Greenhalgh et al., 2016: 418). Greenhalgh and colleagues go so far as to recommend 'co-creation' of initiatives, provided they are both inward and outward facing: inward towards relationships and local circumstances, and outward towards practical-systemic connections and structural (technological, spatial, etc.) dimensions. This point underscores that VRE's focus on *in situ* practice must connect to the implications and consequences of emerging insights and personal learning among stakeholders for managers and policy makers (Iedema and Carroll, 2015). For VRE to hold up as approach, its outcomes will need to be scrutinized from the perspective of what longer-term impacts it has managed to achieve.

In Table 7.1, we set out a range of VRE impacts as these have manifested throughout our projects. In the table, these impacts are arranged from individual to social to practical to systemic impacts. Put differently, the impacts are arranged from 'more cognitive-mental/less easily observable-measurable impact' to 'more material/more observable-measurable impact'.

Table 7.1 Evaluating VRE impacts

Type of impact	Specification
Evidence of participant learning and behaviour change	Participants are enabled to • Recognize that they may have taken their assumptions and habits as given. • Deliberate about their assumptions and habits in acknowledgement that these may need changing. • Become more reflexive and explorative generally in their experience of themselves as people and workers.
Evidence of team conduct change	Teams are enabled to • Scrutinize more systematically, directly and regularly their own practices. • Manifest greater inter- and intra-team flexibility and resilience thanks to regularized feedback and reflexivity. • Redesign care practices and care systems by mobilizing discourses that net in the processual and organizational dimensions of care. • Practice VRE independently as learning and change methodology.
Evidence of practice improvement	Practices display evidence of • Regular times and structured opportunities making feedback and reflexivity 'business as usual'. • Greater practice effectiveness and appropriateness thanks to targeted redesign and strategic adaptation. • Fewer problems and incidents.
Evidence of structures and systems having been impacted	Systems manifest evidence of • Receptiveness to 'innovations from below'. • Enhanced sensitivity to and alignment with constraints and opportunities bearing on actors and practices. • More effective and more organic connections among systems, sub-systems and actors.

VRE's 'impacts' thus range from 'more cognitive-mental/less easily observable-measurable impact' to 'more material/more observable-measurable impact'. We should not call into question 'less easily observable-measurable conduct' as a type of impact, as doing so would rule out participants' 'increased capacity to reflect/rising intelligence/enhanced sense of personal agency' as valid types of healthcare change or improvement outcome. In fact, could it be that the privilege we attribute to provable/measurable kinds of impact has overshadowed less easily measurable manifestations of clinicians' intelligence, sense of agency and learning? Relatedly, could such privilege have served to marginalize participants' learning to act and co-create amidst complexity – both of which are of prime significance to how we take health care into the future?

If the answer is yes to these last two questions, then we have allowed measurement to act as the metaphorical streetlight at night for the drunk who has lost his keys. By elevating measurement to the prime determinant of impact, we risk paying attention to only that area that is illuminated by the street light – to only that which is measurable. We ignore other areas (where the keys may well have been mislaid!) as these remain immeasurable, or 'in the dark'.

VRE takes a different tack by privileging the variety of effects over adherence to measurability, and the constraints and narrowly defined targets that measurement imposes on how we frame care and care improvement.

7.5 AN OVERVIEW OF VRE ACHIEVEMENTS

This section sets out brief reports that summarize VRE achievements accomplished over the years since its inception in 2001. The reports include accounts of achievements in the areas of donor breast milk, patient involvement in infection control, palliative care and critical care handover practices. The reports also detail the relevant evaluation criteria and resulting publications.

7.5.1 Equity in donor breast milk policy (Katherine Carroll)

Donor milk is now made available free of charge to all premature, hospitalized infants in a neonatal intensive care unit (NICU) for the duration of their admission. To date, this accomplishment is the highlight of all the changes made to practice that I have witnessed as a result of working with health professionals, hospital administrators and patients using VRE.

When I arrived in one particular NICU in Denver, Colorado, mothers' own milk was recognized by staff as the gold standard for premature infant feeding. To support exclusive human milk feedings (which dramatically reduce the incidence of the severe disease 'necrotizing enterocolitis' or NEC in premature infants), this NICU's policy was to provide the first 12 ounces (360 mL) of donated breast milk from a human milk bank free of charge when a mother's own milk was unavailable. If the infant required donor milk beyond the first 12 ounces, parents were required to pay for donor milk at the (then) rate of US$4.00/ounce.

During the multidisciplinary video-reflexive session which included me, the researcher, physicians, nurses, dieticians and parent advocates, we viewed ward round footage showing physicians' decision-making and prescribing behaviour in the NICU when infants were facing the end of their free 12 ounces of donor milk. During the reflexivity meeting, NICU staff realized that their donor milk policy needed to change. They realized their current policy of asking parents to pay for donor milk reduced donor milk availability to infants in need and did not align with their goal of exclusive human milk feedings for premature infants.

As a result, the NICU successfully appealed to hospital administrators for the funding of a donor milk programme that would provide donor milk to any infant in need, free of charge, and for the duration of their NICU admission. In addition to the argument of equity in healthcare delivery, the NICU were able to show that any additional costs incurred as a result of providing sufficient donor milk volumes would be more than covered by savings incurred by reducing morbidities and mortalities from the reduction in NEC rates (Carroll, 2014; Iedema and Carroll 2015).

The evaluation criteria (see Table 7.1) that may apply to this case study include the following:

- Participants deliberate about their assumptions and habits in acknowledgement that these may need changing.
- The team intervenes in their existing ways of working in tangible and effective ways.
- Practice displays greater effectiveness and appropriateness thanks to targeted redesign and strategic adaptation.
- The system is susceptible to accountability and responsibility flows impacting on system-level phenomena.

7.5.2 Patient involvement in infection control (Mary Wyer)

A point prevalence survey (a test that establishes the prevalence of infection in a healthcare space) on a surgical ward in a large metropolitan teaching hospital showed higher than average rates of methicillin-resistant *Staphylococcus aureus* acquisition, which placed many patients at greater risk of serious infection. Patients and staff on this ward subsequently took part in a project that used VRE to explore infection risks and design strategies to reduce infection transmission.

In this study, I invited patients to view footage of their own care interactions to identify infection risks, and this led to them coming to new understandings about how safe or unsafe are some infection prevention and control (IPC) practices. For some, this increased their sense of agency, and they developed new strategies for keeping themselves and others safe. For example, one immobile patient asked her nurse for a bottle of alcohol-based hand rub to be placed within reach so that she could wash her hands more regularly. Another saw in the footage the clutter he created with his own belongings and remarked on how this must make it very difficult for cleaners to do their job properly. He decided to bring fewer belongings to hospital on his next visit.

When watching the footage, some patients also became more aware of the roles they had internalized in their interactions with their clinicians and how this affected their abilities to speak up when they felt they were receiving unsafe care. For example, James was at risk of losing his leg due to a foot ulcer that would not heal from a hospital-acquired infection. After watching footage of his own interactions with staff, James came to new understanding of how clinicians can contaminate their gloves before coming to do an invasive procedure on him. He grappled with how he might respond to this next time this happened. Because he felt too embarrassed to ask a staff member to change her gloves, his first plan was to 'accidently' grab the clinician's gloves so that she would be forced to change them.

A few months later when I caught up with James on one of his clinic visits, he told me that while he had never actually grabbed a clinician's gloves, he had devised a new strategy with the community nurses who came to change his dressings and attend to his mother (who also had a wound). He noticed that sometimes the nurses did not change their gloves between doing his dressings and those of his mother. He decided to keep a box of gloves near him and when the nurse was finished doing his mother's dressing, he would hold up the box and say, "Do you need a pair of these?" thus prompting the nurse to change her gloves appropriately before attending to James' wounds (Wyer et al., 2015).

The evaluation criteria that apply to this case study include the following:

- Participants deliberate about existing ways of working, recognizing that their assumptions and habits may need changing.

7.5.3 Creating reflexive space in everyday care (Su-yin Hor)

Two ICUs in a major metropolitan teaching hospital were part of a study exploring the intersections of the built environment, communication and patient safety. Given the broad focus of the study, many themes arose in the first phase of exploration as being of interest to staff in the unit, and also (in my mind) to sociologists and patient safety researchers. For instance, issues of interest included how the multiple instruments attached to patients allowed clinicians to 'monitor' them despite being far away, the use of electronic medical records mediating communication between teams and professionals, the location of large inconvenient pillars blocking views, quiet corridors where staff were isolated in single rooms for long periods of time and so on. All the issues were videoed and discussed in reflexive sessions.

As a novice VRE researcher, trained in ethnographic methods but completely new to the video-reflexive aspects, this level of complexity was daunting. Also, I felt very much the need to contribute something to the unit in exchange for their kind engagement and time given to the project. It did not seem to me to be 'enough' to simply continue with videoing and showing back footage of everyday practices and inviting comment. Later, I understood better the ways in which the VRE process invites participants themselves to focus and drive the change, but for now, my aim was to find a way to contribute, and eventually, after much tearing of hair and gnashing of teeth, it became obvious, through repeated review of my field notes, video footage, interview transcripts and transcripts of reflexive sessions, that there was one issue in particular that participants felt very strongly about – namely, their work being interrupted.

They were angry about the constant interruptions from other staff, loud alarms, phones ringing and basically not being able to concentrate on the important tasks whilst in the unit. At the same time, however, they were also resigned to these interruptions since they were also critical to being able to coordinate action and react quickly to fast-changing patient and ward conditions. Another thing I had noted was that they actually had adopted several strategies to moderate their 'availability' whilst in the ward – such as 'looking busy', getting up and moving around and closing the curtains around a patient's bed.

I put these various facets together in a presentation – with footage of various interruptions captured in the unit, interview quotes and the strategies that they themselves had devised in different situations. I called these 'temporary protected spaces' with 'permeable boundaries', and I was delighted when participants picked these concepts up. They immediately began devising ways in which they could produce temporary but permeable protected spaces for several activities, including the preparation of controlled drugs and the radiology rounds conducted by the intensivists and their team. These strategies were still in place when I visited several years later. The key principle I learnt here is that no matter how much or how little you drive the VRE process, it is always first and foremost about what your participants and collaborators are interested in, and it is their interest that will drive their engagement with and towards practice improvement (Hor et al., 2014).

The evaluation criteria that apply to this case study include the following:

- Participants become more reflexive and explorative generally in their experience of themselves as people and workers.
- Participants deliberate about their assumptions and habits in acknowledgement that these may need changing.

7.5.4 Learning about palliative care (Aileen Collier)

The United Kingdom, Australia and New Zealand policy response to an increasing need for palliative care includes an emphasis that it is not the sole domain of specialists – but rather everybody's business. This response assumes a shared understanding of palliative care, and of role and task divisions among and between specialists and generalists. Disparate interpretations are common and can give rise to considerable tensions (Gott et al., 2011).

Our project, titled 'Brilliance in Evidence-Based Palliative Care', combined positive organizational scholarship in healthcare and VRE to focus on positive practices of community palliative care teams in two states of Australia. Dr. Ann Dadich along with Michael Hodgins carried out fieldwork along with co-researcher clinicians in New South Wales (in Australia) and Dr. Aileen Collier in the state of South Australia. The study aimed to better understand the conditions that produced 'brilliant' community palliative care. Although focused on the positive, this project did not ignore problems and also identified the areas of improvement.

At the beginning of a VRE project like this, one is never quite sure where the research might lead. Perhaps because of the project's open-ended focus, in the beginning staff was highly suspicious. Had someone sent us for surveillance purposes? And how on earth were we going to video in the home of someone requiring palliative care?

VRE accomplishments are sometimes much less about outcomes in the way they are conventionally thought of and 'measured', and much more about strengthening people's agency and relationships. It involves building the kinds of 'affective spheres' that Iedema and Carroll (2015) describe. This was very much evident within the Brilliance project. Staff came to know and trust that our way of 'being' researchers and 'doing' research was quite different to more conventional research. The project moved individuals, clinical teams and patient and families to act in new ways.

For example, in New South Wales (Australia), the generalist community nursing team, to a large extent and historically, did not invest in providing palliative care despite it being a growing component of their role. Rather, they tended to defer to their specialist palliative care nurse colleagues. In turn, this frustrated the small team of three specialist palliative care nurses who saw their role as supporting and building the capacity of the generalist community nursing colleagues rather than just providing direct care.

As a result of 'seeing' their own and other clinicians' practices through VRE and interrogating these practices in reflexive sessions, both teams better understood their respective roles. Subsequently, the generalist community nurses became more appreciative of the palliative care dimensions of their own role. As both generalist nurses and specialist nurses worked alongside researchers, filming, editing and presenting the project to inside and outsider stakeholders, team relationships developed and generalist community nurses became more committed to enacting palliative care. As the area manager for Palliative Care & Service Development of the Local Health District stated in an email (Dadich et al., 2018; Collier et al., (accepted for publication):

> You, Ann, Michael are really pioneers in helping us to look differently at what we do, how we do it & why. I love that you are influencing so many & bringing them on this research journey. It's creating enthusiasm, renewed love & respect of our profession/speciality, & reinvigorating the word 'teamwork'.

The evaluation criteria that apply to this case study include the following:

- Participants become more reflexive and explorative generally in their experience of themselves as people and workers.
- Teams scrutinize more systematically, directly and regularly their own practices.

7.5.5 Development of an ambulance-to-emergency department handover protocol (Rick Iedema)

This project was initiated to systematize the ambulance-to-emergency department (ED) handover process in New South Wales, Australia. The project addressed health department concerns that handover practices between ambulance and ED staff was suboptimal, and that incidents occurred as a result. Instead of prescribing the use of a particular protocol, the NSW Department of Health agreed to the logic of VRE and allowed ambulance and ED staff to co-design their own protocol.

Ambulance officers' and ED clinicians' involvement in the project was secured on the basis that this VRE study, its success and outcomes would be entirely dependent on their participation. VRE ensured that paramedics and clinicians had an opportunity to analyze their own practices, share their sense of accomplishment about being able to carry off complex kinds of work in challenging circumstances, align their understandings about current problems, challenges and information needs and, collectively redesign alternative ways of working and communicating.

Ambulance paramedics and ED staff were videoed while conducting handovers before any other intervention occurred. Footage of 73 handovers was collected in this way and analyzed. The analysis included listing the individual clinical information components that made up existing handovers, non-verbal communication (eye contact, body distance and movements) and the duration of the handover patterns (including triage and resuscitation bay handover). This data was correlated with paramedics' levels of expertise and the disease severity of their patients to uncover regularities.

The footage and analyses were shared with both ambulance and ED staff, and a consensus was drawn up about the things that both professional groups felt needed to change. This consensus statement came to be called IMIST-AMBO, where I stands for 'identification', M for 'mechanism/medical complaint', I for 'injuries/information relating to the complaint', S for 'signs', T for 'treatment and trends', A for 'allergies', M for 'medication', B for 'background history' and O for 'other information'. The protocol further specifies bodily behaviours (eye contact and body distance) and contextual conditions (a space of non-interruption and general attentiveness).

Analysis of video footage of 74 pre- and 63 post-intervention handovers, combined with results from ED staff questionnaires, points to an improvement in communication between ambulance paramedics and ED clinicians following the introduction of the IMIST-AMBO protocol. Improvement was evident from the video data analysis on the following fronts: a more consistent ordering of the information components, a greater frequency of the necessary information components, and reduction in information repetition and asking of questions, possibly suggesting better comprehension and retention of information by recipients, and eye contact between paramedics and ED clinicians associating with the reduction in handover duration, intimating that eye contact may improve the efficiency of information exchange.

Following this, at hospital site 1, 60 clinicians and 118 paramedics were trained in the new protocol. This targeted training and feedback took place over 3 weeks. The same process unfolded at hospital site 2 and lasted 2 weeks. During this period, 48 clinicians and 102 paramedics were trained at site 2, or a total of 150 staff. A further 45 paramedic educators were also trained in the protocol. The grand total of staff trained across both sites was 373 over a total of 5 weeks. The number 373 constitutes over 10% of the total number of paramedics currently employed in New South Wales. IMIST-AMBO has since been adopted in various sites around the world, including in the United States and New Zealand (Iedema et al., 2012).

The evaluation criteria that apply to this case study include the following:

- Actors deliberate about their assumptions and habits in acknowledgement that these may need changing.
- Teams scrutinize more systematically and directly their own practices.
- Teams manifest greater inter- and intra-team flexibility and resilience thanks to feedback and reflexivity.
- Teams redesign care practices and care systems by mobilizing discourses that net in the processual and organizational dimensions of care.
- Practices manifest higher levels of effectiveness and appropriateness thanks to targeted redesign and strategic adaptation.
- The system (of state-wide ambulance to ED handover and paramedic training) shows receptiveness to 'innovations from below'.

7.5.6 VRE is there to stay ... (Jessica Mesman)

When their lives are seriously at risk, newborn babies are admitted to the neonatology ward. Very ill babies end up in the NICU of this ward. Their vulnerability calls for maximum support of their vital functions and adherence to hygiene rules to prevent infections.

My collaboration with the Neonatology ward of the Maastricht University Medical Centre started in the early 1990s as part of my PhD project on uncertainty in critical care. In the mid-2000s, I studied patient safety in order to focus on practitioners' existing practices and illuminate or 'exnovate' the robustness of practices. Using this lens, I was again able to collaborate with the same NICU.

While I was engaged in this project, I was hosted by Rick Iedema at his research centre in Sydney, Australia, and I worked alongside his PhD student Katherine Carroll on their Australian Research Council-funded project on clinical handover. It was during this period that I learned about VRE. Returning to the Netherlands, I showed the management of the NICU this new tool for research *and* practice improvement. Their response was very positive, and it was decided to use VRE on the ward.

For NICU staff, it was important to focus on infection prevention and catheter-related bloodstream infections in particular. I started VRE on the NICU in the role of what we now identify as a clinalyst (Iedema and Carroll 2011). Although in close collaboration with the clinicians, I was the one who filmed, edited the footage, organized the meetings and chaired the reflexive sessions. However, my position at the university involved a lot of teaching commitments, and this limited my ability to do research. During my weeks of teaching, VRE activities on the NICU came to a complete standstill. This frustrated both the clinicians and me. To solve this problem, I trained a small group of clinicians – a so-called video team – to take over my role. This led to my gradually becoming obsolete.

Since 2011, this ward has been using VRE without an external facilitator. VRE is now a structural part of their practice. The meetings are attended by both physicians and nurses. All clinicians can use their own experience and expertise in these reflexive meetings. Due to the team's ongoing discussions during their reflexive meetings, staff has found it easier to address issues and problems during their actual performance of NICU procedures. Now nurses have the opportunity to discuss even challenging issues with the doctors as they can refer to their previous reflexive discussions. On basis of these discussions, several protocols have been adjusted. In these instances, discussions have resulted in shared agreement about the importance of making a particular change to the protocol. Many other changes have been made over the years. In almost all cases, the changes were small, but it is the detail that counts, especially for patient safety and NICU infection prevention.

Over the years, this NICU has received two awards for VRE as best practice. For me their biggest achievement is the fact that they are able to maintain VRE as being a part of their professional ecology. This is remarkable considering the plethora of safety and quality projects that tend to compete for clinicians' attention. Many projects come and fade away. This NICU has chosen VRE over other forms of improvement and has been able to make it a sustainable part of their everyday work (Mesman, 2015).

The evaluation criteria that apply to this case study include the following:

- Actors deliberate about their assumptions and habits in acknowledgement that these may need changing.
- Teams practice VRE independently as learning and change methodology.
- Practices manifest higher levels of effectiveness and appropriateness thanks to targeted redesign and strategic adaptation.
- The system (of neonatal service provision) shows receptiveness to 'innovations from below'.

7.6 METHODS OF VRE EVALUATION

The above accounts setting out achievements make clear that evaluating VRE projects involves an opportunistic element: anything that points to the possibility of having improved practice may be consolidated into the overall assessment of our VRE project. Thus, we harness off-the-cuff comments, chance observations, thank-you emails and people's impressions to demonstrate that our project paid off. Methodologically then, the evaluation of VRE is an agnostic practice. We may draw on surveys, before-and-after footage, interviews and focus groups, as well as on *ad hoc* remarks and chance experiences.

This does not mean that VRE has not been evaluated more 'rigourously'. The IMIST-AMBO study involved a systematic evaluation of post-training handovers. As reported earlier, videoed evidence revealed that paramedics handed patients over using their protocol more often and for more information than was the case before the training. A recently concluded project on the impact of VRE in the area of IPC found that the video-reflexive sessions coincided with a considerable drop in hospital-acquired infections among patients (Gilbert et al., in preparation).

That said, the evaluation of interventions that tackle complex aspects of care will always be challenged when it comes to proving their impact. This challenge becomes more acute when we move closer towards the front-line of care, that is, the zone of maximum complexity (Iedema, 2015). This challenge does not necessarily call for more rigourous project designs or more systematic measurements. We would argue the contrary. Care improvement is and remains a complex affair, and it will only become more complex in the future. Our principal challenge therefore is not measurement and evidence of past impact, but learning and the production of ongoing impact amidst complex circumstances.

7.7 CONCLUSION

This chapter has addressed the vexed issue of how to evaluate VRE initiatives, and it has proposed a range of evaluation criteria. Evaluating VRE initiatives can be challenging because this practice may need to rely on unconventional resources (besides measurements) and multiple kinds of evidence (potentially including narratives, videos, off-the-cuff statements and corridor conversations). Given VRE is interested not principally in knowledge about the complexities with which it engages, and targets learning that enables actors to meet the demands of complex practices and systems more effectively, VRE relies on impact testimonials and empirical analyses of *in situ* practice that bear out or *model* such learning.

For their part, VRE's achievements have ranged from enabling more preterm infants to receive donor breast milk, to patients becoming explicit about their experience of in-hospital infections, patients speaking about the quality of their end of life, teams enabled to strengthen their 'teamness', ambulance and ED staff being enabled to coordinate their information exchanges and communication more generally and a neonatal team adopting VRE as an in-house improvement approach. These are but selected examples of VRE impact. Collectively, they point towards VRE providing a powerful resource for bringing participants together in the face of complex challenges, providing the means to enhancing people's intelligence and insight into how to act amidst complexity.

REFERENCES

Bate P and Robert G. (2007) *Bringing User Experience to Healthcare Improvement: The Concepts, Methods and Practices of Experience-Based Design.* Oxford/Seattle, WA: Radcliffe.

Bosk CL, Dixon-Woods M, Goeschel C, et al. (2009) The art of medicine: Reality check for checklists. *Lancet* 374: 444–445.

Carroll K, Iedema R and Kerridge R. (2008) Reshaping ICU ward round practices using video reflexive ethnography. *Qualitative Health Research* 18: 380–390.

Carroll, K. (2014). Body dirt or liquid gold? How the safety of donor human milk is constructed for use in neonatal intensive care. *Social Studies of Science*, 44(3), 466–485.

Collier, A., Hodgins, M., Crawford,G., et al. (accepted for publication) Bringing brilliance to light in home-based palliative care: A video reflexive ethnography study. *Palliative Medicine*.

Chatterji AP. (2001) Postcolonial research as relevant practice. *Tamara: Journal of Critical Postmodern Organization Science* 13 https://tamarajournal.com/index.php/tamara/article/view/37/32

Dadich, A., Collier, A., Hodgins, M., et al. (2018). Using positive organizational scholarship in healthcare and video reflexive ethnography to examine positive deviance to new public management in healthcare. Qualitative Health Research. doi:10.1177/1049732318759492.

Gawande A. (2011) *Checklist Manifesto*. London: Profile Books.

Gilbert L, O'Sullivan M, Dempsey K, et al. (in preparation) Whatever it takes: A prospective intervention study, using videoreflexive methods (VRM) and enhanced conventional infection prevention and control, to reduce MRSA transmission in two surgical wards.

Gordon L, Rees C, Ker J, et al. (2016) Using video-reflexive ethnography to capture the complexity of leadership enactment in the healthcare workplace. *Advances in Health Science Education*. doi:10.1007/s10459-10016-19744-z.

Greenhalgh T, Jackson C, Shaw S, et al. (2016) Achieving research impact through co-creation in community-based health services: Literature review and case study. *Milbank Quarterly* 94: 392–429.

Gott, M., Seymour, J., Ingleton, C.,et al. (2011). 'That's part of everybody's job': the perspectives of health care staff in England and New Zealand on the meaning and remit of palliative care. *Palliative Medicine*, 232–241.

Hor S, Iedema R and Manias E. (2014) Creating spaces in intensive care for safe communication: A video-reflexive ethnographic study. *BMJ Quality & Safety* 23: 1007–1013.

Iedema R. (2015) *Three ACI-Sponsored Initiatives: Lessons for System-Wide Change*. Sydney: Agency for Clinical Innovation (NSW Ministry of Health).

Iedema, R. and Carroll, K. (2015). Research as affect-sphere: Towards spherogenics. *Emotion Review*, 7(1), 67–72.

Iedema R, Ball C, Daly B, et al. (2012) Design and trial of a new ambulance-to-emergency department handover protocol: 'IMIST-AMBO'. *BMJ Quality & Safety* 21: 627–633.

Iedema R and Carroll K. (2015) Research as affect-sphere: Towards spherogenics. *Emotion Review* 7: 1–7.

Iedema, R., and Carroll, K. (2011). The Clinalyst: Institutionalizing reflexive space to realize safety and flexible systematization in health care. *Journal of Organizational Change Management*, 24(2), 175–190.

Iedema R, Merrick E and Kerridge R, et al. (2009) 'Handover – Enabling Learning in Communication for Safety' (HELiCS): A report on achievements at two hospital sites. *Medical Journal of Australia* 190: S133–S136.

King DK, Glasgow RE, and Leeman-Castillo B. (2010) Reaiming RE-AIM: Using the model to plan, implement, and evaluate the effects of environmental change approaches to enhancing population health. *American Journal of Public health* 100: 2076–2084.

Medical Research Council (UK). (2006) *Developing and Evaluating Complex Interventions*. London: Medical Research Council (UK).

Mertens DM. (2009) *Transformative Research and Evaluation*. New York: Guildford Press.

Mesman, J. (2015) Boundary-spanning engagements on a neonatal ward: A collaborative entanglement between clinicians and researchers. In: Collaboration across Health Research and Care. Penders, B., Vermeulen, N., and Parker, J. (eds.) Aldershot: Ashgate Publishing Ltd: 171–194.

Mitchell S. (2009) *Unsimple Truths: Science, Complexity and Policy*. Chicago, IL: Chicago University Press.

Neuwirth EB, Bellows J, Jackson AH, et al. (2012) How kaiser permanente uses video ethnography of patients for quality improvement. *Health Affairs* 31: 1244–1250.

Ovretveit J. (2011) Understanding the conditions for improvement: Research to discover which context influences affect improvement success. *BMJ Quality & Safety* 20 (Supp 1): i18–i23.

Pawson R and Tilley N. (1997) *Realistic Evaluation*. London: Sage.

Wyer, M., Jackson, D, Iedema, R., et al. (2015). Involving patients in understanding hospital infection control using visual methods. *Journal of Clinical Nursing*, 24(11–12), 1718–1729.

Wyer M, Iedema R, Hor S, et al. (2017) Patient involvement can affect clinicians' perspectives and practices of infection prevention and control: A 'post-qualitative' study using video-reflexive ethnography. *International Journal of Qualitative Research Methods* 16: 1–10.

8

Publishing VRE studies

8.1 INTRODUCTION

After being immersed in the richness of fieldwork, engaging with research participants and other stakeholders, collating, viewing and editing video footage and enjoying the fruitful collaborations that make tangible changes and contributions to healthcare delivery, it is time to take yet another step: disseminating your video-reflexive ethnography (VRE) research. This may take the form of publishing, presenting it at a conference, integrating it into health service policy or healthcare professional training. Besides letting others know about your VRE project's achievements, these are also ways of evaluating, confirming and increasing the impact of your project by sharing it with audiences beyond the immediate project team. In this chapter, we will take you through various considerations involved in translating your VRE study into written and spoken outputs. We will help you to consider what you and your participants may like to share from your VRE project with broader audiences. We will also consider the aspects of VRE work that do not lend themselves well to being published.

First, we commence this chapter by examining common issues associated with publishing VRE research for academic purposes or in academic venues such as book chapters and peer-reviewed journals. In this section, we touch on encouraging the VRE researcher to consider important ethical, theoretical and practical issues that need to be conveyed in published work, such as debates around representation of people and organizational processes in visual data, the use of text versus pictures in publications, authorship and participant or site anonymity. For those who have worked with visual methods, many of our considerations will have aspects in common with those governing the publication of visual methods research.

Second, wrapping up a VRE study often involves more than the dissemination of findings through publication and presentation. It may also mean implementing findings from reflexivity sessions or ensuring that the new VRE skills are taught such that they become part of the clinical team's improvement repertoire. One way of doing this is through the production of a handbook and instructional video that is made available to the team, or by training team members in VRE (Mesman, 2015).

8.2 A BREADTH OF PUBLICATION OPTIONS

More than 150 articles and book chapters have been published on VRE, attracting over 1,000 citations. In these publications, the VRE methodology may feature as the primary methodology (Iedema et al., 2010; Iedema and Carroll, 2015; Stone et al., 2015; Collier et al., 2016; Collier and Wyer, 2016) or as a sub-component of mixed-methods empirical studies (Lammer, 2009; Hor et al., 2017). Alternatively, your publication may foreground service provider and service user concerns (Carroll, 2009; Forsyth, 2009; Van Helmond et al., 2015). It may report on how video enabled you and participants to learn about patients' or health professionals' expertise (Collier and Wyer, 2016), or enhance their communication, and therefore the quality and safety of health care (Iedema, 2011; Hor et al., 2014). You may also decide to publish about pragmatic ethnographic interventions (Grant and Luxford, 2009; Carroll and Mesman, 2011). Or you may discuss the more theoretical and philosophical bases of research, such as how VRE shifts our attention from prioritizing 'matters of fact' towards negotiating 'matters of concern' (Hor and Iedema, 2015).

Publication avenues for VRE reports include clinical journals such as those pertaining to medicine and nursing (e.g., *Journal of Clinical Nursing*, *BMJ Quality & Safety*), social science journals such as those in sociology and organizational studies (e.g., *Sociology of Health & Illness*, *Organization Studies*), interdisciplinary journals such as those in the broad area of health and health services research (e.g., *Health*, *Social Science & Medicine*) and methodology journals such as those that focus on qualitative and visual methodologies (e.g., *Qualitative Health Research*). Qualitative methods journals may at times accept special issues on how VRE as methodology itself has advanced (e.g., the special issue on VRE published in 2009 in the *International Journal of Multiple Research Approaches*) or on how VRE informs and intersects with other collaborative or related visual methods (Dieckmann et al., 2017).

VRE publications may emphasize the success of the VRE methodology itself and highlight the innovative and participative ways in which it draws on visualizations of practice, visual feedback or the expertise of participants (Iedema et al., 2006). VRE publications may also report on our philosophical reflections on the connections among visual feedback, reflexivity and the becoming-more-intelligent of people's taken-as-given habits and otherwise unquestioned assumptions (Iedema and Bezemer, under review). Publications may also describe how VRE has made a difference to people's experiences of healthcare delivery (Carroll et al., 2008; Carroll, 2009; Forsyth, 2009; Grant and Luxford, 2009).

VRE publications may further focus on the substantive changes VRE has made to a particular group's practice (Iedema et al., 2009) or to a profession's training curriculum and relevant policy reform (Iedema et al., 2012). Publications may report too on the role VRE has played in the learning by clinical or academic staff about a particular healthcare area, such as maternity care (Leap et al., 2009). In all, there are many angles and opportunities for researchers and clinicians to publish about their VRE studies. While such publications are likely to be somewhat unconventional in their reliance on multiple approaches to evaluation and data presentation, there are many avenues enabling us to explore and register the contributions of VRE on healthcare practice.

Scholars, clinicians and other users of VRE are not limited to publishing in academic journals. VRE has also been published in book chapters (Iedema, 2011; Mesman, 2011; Hor and Iedema, 2015; Sormani et al., 2017), as PhD theses (Forsyth, 2006; Carroll, 2009; Collier, 2013; McLeod, 2017; Wyer, 2017; Lenne, 2018), as scholarly books such as the present book, as full-length monographs (Iedema et al., 2013) and as videos and documentaries (e.g., the video produced to accompany the 2008 HELiCS booklet; the documentaries produced by Dr. Verena Thomas in collaboration with villagers in Papua New Guinea: *Yumi Piksa* and *Komuniti Tok Piksa*). By briefly detailing the scope and reach of these publications, we hope to have conveyed that there are many options and routes for publishing VRE research, and myriad ways of tackling issues raised by VRE in your projects.

8.3 WHY PUBLISH VRE PROJECTS?

It is invariably rewarding to work with clinical teams, patients, and their families and be party to how they are enabled to make tangible changes to healthcare delivery and clinical experiences. For some, VRE may be rewarding enough to leave it there. The Utrecht clinical handover study led by Professor Cor Kalkman in the Netherlands, for example, achieved remarkable outcomes across several hospitals, but these have not been widely reported (Iedema et al., 2013). Most likely, this is because publishing VRE research and practice improvement interventions is not straightforward, particularly for those who may work outside of academia or in specialist-clinical research institutions. You may not be accustomed to the genre of scholarly writing or the cross-disciplinary orientation of VRE studies. Clinicians may feel that the qualitative research, theoretical or methodology journals that may accept VRE reports are too different from how they have been inducted into thinking about and writing up research.

Publishing means engaging in a global (international) dialogue about your experiences and findings resulting from using VRE. Such dialogue enriches VRE theory and methodology, enabling other researchers and clinicians to benefit from VRE developments and innovations. Publishing may have a personal benefit too, as it helps build one's own credibility as a VRE researcher. This, in turn, assists you in fostering relations with future stakeholders, VRE collaborators or field sites in which you hope to deploy VRE. Given VRE is a developing endeavour, there are numerous theoretical, methodological and ethical–legal aspects to be explored.

As a social scientist, publishing VRE research in a clinical journal (as opposed to a social science journal) may assist you (and other social scientists who may use your work) in developing future collaborations with healthcare professionals and institutions. It is not uncommon (as we advised in previous chapters) for VRE researchers to bring to initial meetings with potential collaborators, published VRE studies showing evidence of practice improvement, engagement with similar staff, uptake by prominent organizations (Carroll et al., 2018) or more general systems-level achievements (Iedema et al., 2012). In our experience, publications contribute to enabling VRE to be accepted as a credible methodology in the clinical space. Being able to refer to the key aspects of VRE theory and method in existing publications may mollify those who are new to VRE, including people with roles in funding bodies, ethics committees, healthcare improvement agencies or healthcare service boards.

8.4 ACADEMIC PUBLISHING OF YOUR VRE PROJECT

Previous chapters have already detailed at length the four guiding theoretical principles of VRE: exnovation, collaboration, reflexivity and care. While VRE is principally concerned to register practical impact, its processes are guided by these principles. The effects of these processes may be illuminated by referring to people's comments about the VRE process, to before-and-after footage (rendered as stills or included as online video files) of *in situ* practice or to evidence derived (in visual or spoken form) from reflexive sessions. It is a common critique, however, that visual methods research tends to be published in primarily textual form (Mannay, 2016).

In the case of VRE, the moving image tends to be presented as the method's defining characteristic, alongside collaboration with participants and their reflexivity and its tangible impacts on people, their teams, practices and systems. It is therefore natural that visual data be included in some form in publications. Visuals are important for drawing readers' attention to: (i) the often unnoticed complexity of care delivery practices; (ii) the moving image's ability to elicit key learnings among researchers, clinicians, patients and families and (iii) the fact that visual evidence (in contrast to linguistic or numerical evidence) functions well as portrayal of changes in self-identity, team interaction and/or healthcare practices as a result of deploying VRE. To include such visuals in publications, you may need to experiment with turning video footage into stills or drawings, or you may want to inquire into whether the journal accepts supplementary video files which it hosts online.

Regardless of the *type* of footage (whether it features patients and family members receiving care from clinical staff, or clinical staff reviewing videos of themselves in a reflexive session) and the *form* of footage (still frames or cartoon drawings or moving images), a common set of questions will need to be asked of the footage, of participants, of yourself as a researcher and perhaps even of the institutions involved before selecting the visuals for publication. These questions primarily relate to the VRE guiding principle of 'care' (ensuring the psychological safety (Edmondson, 1999) of participants). Such care is to be carried out by ensuring appropriate or required levels of participant anonymity and institutional confidentiality. How to realize appropriate levels of care and participant safety will further depend on the publication venue, any human research ethics requirements and data use agreements you've struck with your participants and organizations. For instance, with regard to publication venue and human research ethics committee requirements, some VRE projects may only have permission to publish visual images for internal team use only, whereas other projects may enjoy broader publication and international dissemination opportunities.

With regard to requirements around anonymity and confidentiality, different considerations and motivations may shape how these are satisfied in your paper. For instance, foregrounding the collaborative principle will produce publications that prioritize giving voice to participants. Consider in this regard how Foster discusses her work promoting the interests of working-class mothers in the North West of London:

> Amongst the participants themselves, the work produced led to discussions about how poor working-class women are viewed by wider society. However, I feel that there was a potential to take these discussions to a larger audience, using the videos as a tool to generate a wider debate on representations of poor, working-class women. In future research employing participatory video, I would consider building in means of dissemination to a much more sizeable audience at the beginning of a project, making links with local organisations and media in order to gain access to a wider public.
>
> *(Foster, 2009: 243)*

Foster acknowledges that preserving people's anonymity prevented her from generating 'wider debate' about participants' working-class circumstances. For her next project, she writes, she would 'consider building in means of dissemination to a much more sizable audience at the beginning of the project'. To do so, she would need a broader remit for her project's consent processes and for her use of project data in publications.

If participants are willing to be featured in such publications, and if they consent to your use of video data in which they feature, you will have to address the question of what boundaries to place around their representation. In some cases, you may find that your participants remain protective of their identities and appearances, and are reluctant to sign over the right to you to publish visuals of them at work. In other cases, as Aileen Collier found, you may encounter participants who regard you as the vehicle for disseminating their message to the world (Collier, 2013).

In most cases, participants may be happy to negotiate with you about the best approach to the use of their visuals. This may include deciding on specific visuals that they are happy to have published, following particular renderings (pixellation, blurring, cartoonizing) to ensure their anonymity, or the substitution of authentic footage with videoed re-enactments of relevant scenes and events, or restricted types of publication (e.g., social science journals only) or specific kinds of presentation (specific conferences only). You may consider the use of comics to represent visual data (Brossard and Sapin-Leduc, 2017) or deploy specialized text types to do so, including the letter format (Carroll, 2015), or a poem (Mannay, 2016).

In writing this book, we collectively pondered the question of whether and how to publish visual data from our own research projects. The complex issues we faced in considering the inclusion of VRE video data in this book are here set out as a case study. The case study aims to convey how we deliberated and decided these issues (see Box 8.1).

BOX 8.1: What video data shall we include in this book?

In discussing which visual data we would include in this book, we all agreed to review the video data that we had archived from various VRE projects and consider which of these could be used for publication. We asked ourselves the following questions:

- What understandings do human research ethics committees, participating institutions and individual participants have about where and how visual data from past VRE projects will be disseminated?
- What formal human research ethics committee approvals, consents and agreements do we have for sharing existing video data for the purposes of publishing a methodological book?
- If there is visual data that we consider amenable to publication, to what extent will that visual data need to be anonymized?

We also needed to interrogate how video data may be shared as part of the publication of a text-based book. If the video data were to be handed over to the publisher and hosted on the publishers' website, what would that mean for copyright, ownership and control over the visual data? Relatedly, what chances might there be for visual data to be downloaded and used in unplanned ways by people not originally involved in the relevant project, project publications, the present book or the publishing company?

In the past, we have relied on ethics approval, consent and media release procedures for how we approached the editing of video footage. Thus, we have turned footage into sequences of still frames using pixellation and other kinds of rendering to ensure de-identification (Iedema et al., 2006; Iedema, 2011). Should we adopt those strategies here? Upon reviewing these questions individually and as a group, we realized that our retrospectively constructed video data arising from our various VRE studies could not always ethically and legally be shared as part of the publication of this book as video data per se.

This is particularly the case now that the General Data Protection Regulation (GDPR) is in force across the European continent (European Union, 2018). The GDPR sets strict rules around the reach of people's consent and advises that if a particular future use of data was not envisaged, it cannot be assumed that such use is legitimate. The GDPR is not designed to limit data use however, but to ensure that any data use aligns with the original consent obtained. We acknowledge therefore, as did Foster above, that in our forthcoming VRE projects, we should deploy more forward-looking and more general consent procedures enabling us to gain permission for the use of video footage (as clips, stills, cartoons and the like) for not-as-yet conceived but related (in content) and relevant (in spirit) projects.

Building on Foster's reflections and on our own thoughts around visually illustrating this book, we advise you to think ahead to the time when you would like to use video data in publications and presentations. In doing so, it is important to remember that your obligations towards human research ethics committees and towards institutional stakeholders will continue to determine decisions about the dissemination of video data. For that reason, your ethical and institutional approvals should make reference to whether and how visual evidence may be used for dissemination going into the future.

In offering this advice however, we also acknowledge that determining in advance what you would like to do with visual data may not always be possible. As discussed in previous chapters, VRE may take projects in directions that were unimaginable at the time the project was described for ethics committees or developed with stakeholders and participants (Wills et al., 2016). As Wills and colleagues put it,

> stringent rules about the governance of a study are sometimes inappropriate and often impossible to apply. This is partly due to the impossibility of setting *a-priori* conditions about what participation will involve and what images might be filmed or photographed in a study.
>
> *(Wills et al., 2016: 481)*

Exemplifying this, clinician-participants may find that a portion of visual data is ideally suited to patient education and, for that reason, may request *post hoc* to amend human research ethics requirements or renegotiate agreements about visual data dissemination with participants (Wills et al., 2016). Or it may be that an infection control professional finds that a portion of visual data turns out to be a perfect resource for sparking constructive conversations among clinicians about infection control. Or a national quality and safety agency may decide that particular video clips are useful for enriching staff presentations at national and international conferences and policy forums. Each of these kinds of situations creates opportunities for a much wider dissemination of project outcomes and their visual data than you may have envisaged, and they require you to make decisions about such unexpected opportunities that respect ethics committees' edicts, participants' rights and preferences and VRE's commitment to care.

We compiled a list of questions that you should ask about how the visual data is going to be used over and above the reflexive meetings (Table 8.1). These questions are intended to sensitize you to the risks that may be present when publishing visual resources that have the potential to identify participants and sites.

8.5 CONTROLLING OTHERS' ACCESS TO YOUR VIDEO DATA

Digital images can be shared 'instantly and globally via the Internet, often beyond the control of the researcher' (Cox et al., 2014: 9). For this reason, in 2010 one of the keynote speakers at the third International Visual Methods Conference in

Table 8.1 Questions relating to the dissemination of visual data

Questions relating to	Questions
Ethics committees' decisions and approvals	Has your human research ethics committee or institutional review board granted approval for the dissemination of visual data? What level/type of dissemination has been approved?
The modality of representation	Will video (moving image) data be shared in publications, posters or presentations, or will a series of stills be used instead?
	What degree of identifiability is the visual data allowed?
Control over the medium of publishing/dissemination	Who will host the data for publishing? Will it be the publisher's website, a video-sharing platform like YouTube or Vimeo, or your own project or institution's website?
	What does your publication plan mean for control over the availability and use of images and their copyright?
	If material is published by the publisher of books or journals on behalf of the author, is copyright retained by the authors, the health service or the participants, or transferred to the publisher?
Individual participants	Will you be able to follow up with participants once data has been collected to re-consent them regarding data collected and the plans for dissemination?
	Will participants have an opportunity to view and approve the footage before it was made publically available?
	Has a media release form been signed by participants featured in the footage?
	Do participants who feature in the footage agree to it being made available online?
	Did the participants think through and understand the consequences of this material being made available online? How can this understanding be tested?
Institutional stakeholders	What legal and formal agreements with hospitals or universities govern the ownership, publication and sharing of video data?
	Are identifying features of the health service such as logos, spaces and signs taken out or obscured?

(Continued)

Table 8.1 (*Continued*) Questions relating to the dissemination of visual data

Questions relating to	Questions
Degree of identifiability of participants and sites	(To what extent) will participants' faces be blurred/pixelated?
	(To what extent) will the visuals as a whole be cartoonized (cf. some of the images used in Chapters 1 and 5)?
	(To what extent) will participants have their voices changed?

BOX 8.2: Containing access to visual data

'I had the experience where someone videoed my whole conference presentation – with patient footage – without me knowing. Someone told me afterwards and I had to chase the person down. She said she was going to use it as educational material for her staff. I asked her to delete it – and just had to trust that she did. My supervisor and I agreed that we'd send an email to the conference organisers and ask for the matter to be followed up. They sent an email back saying that the person assured them that the recording had been deleted.'

Wellington, Aotearoa New Zealand, requested explicitly at the beginning of her lecture that the audience not use their mobile phones to take pictures of her slides or record the presentation in any way. In Box 8.2, Mary Wyer recounts her experience of having her presentation (including clips) filmed without her knowledge.

Another issue to consider is when conferences ask you to upload your presentation and clips on their computers. Is their practice to delete all these files afterwards? Or is their practice to publish your presentation on their site? In these instances, you may need to require the organizers to remove the video clips and replace them with a slide saying 'video removed for privacy reasons'. Also think of instances where you are asked to present a lecture as part of a course and you have to copy your presentation to the lecture room's computer. You will have to remember to delete your file(s) or wait until an appropriate time to move your presentation to trash and delete the trash.

While it makes sense for you to maintain control over your video data, could there be any adverse implications for restricting public access or ensuring participants' anonymity? Some scholars argue that restricting access and maintaining anonymity risks 'dehumanising participants' (Cox et al., 2014). In a similar vein, Mannay refers to an 'impasse' that many collaborative and participatory visual researchers have had to confront in this regard:

... even if images are successfully anonymized, acts to disguise images can be seen as tantamount to silencing the voice of research participants. This is particularly problematic where researchers invest in the epistemological approaches predicated on giving 'voice'. In contrast to an emphasis on 'protection' through anonymization … collaborative projects in which participants are visible and recognisable is an alternative approach to ethical social research.

(Mannay, 2016: 110)

Mannay (2016: 110) does concede however that 'some participants may want some level of anonymity and some topics may be particularly sensitive; and in such cases being visible and recognisable may not be practical, possible or ethical'. There is a tension then between research that seeks to foreground previously unheard and unseen aspects of social life, and the obligation to ensure anonymity and confidentiality.

In what follows, we consider two examples of VRE projects where participants have expressly wanted to be recognized in broadly disseminated footage (Box 8.3 and Box 8.4). Both are examples of initiatives that allowed wide dissemination to external audiences of video clips featuring clear images of VRE participants. These two examples highlight how participants' being clearly visible *and* recognizable can add to the impact of how we disseminate VRE experiences and findings.

The first example is drawn from the work of Jessica Mesman (see Box 8.3). This example makes apparent that the clips in question harboured a special emotional intensity. They engendered special resonances for audiences and exerted greater influence.

BOX 8.3: An example of a project allowing for the dissemination of fully identifying visual data

In her work on positive approaches to researching patient safety, Jessica Mesman routinely presents identifiable VRE data to audiences of health professionals and academics. Some of her data features a neonatal intensive care unit (NICU) team in the Netherlands practising the 'planned obsolescence' model of doing VRE. In this model of doing VRE, the researcher hands VRE over to the NICU team who themselves and independently continue the VRE methodology as part of their approach to quality and safety (Carroll and Mesman 2018). The NICU team feels very proud of their accomplishment, and rather than requesting Mesman to blur their faces, the team uses fully identifiable footage featuring the NICU clinical team meeting to review video ethnographic footage of their own practices. In fact, they favoured this footage being shown publicly with their institution's logos being visible, ensuring their unit and hospital are remembered as being unique in adopting VRE to optimize local care practices.

The second example of wide dissemination to external audiences of video clips featuring clear images of VRE participants pertains to the involvement of participants in the publication and presentation of VRE research, which we turn to now.

8.6 INVOLVING PARTICIPANTS IN THE PUBLICATION AND PRESENTATION OF VRE RESEARCH

You may want to push participants' involvement in VRE projects one step further again. In Box 8.4, we present a case study describing Mary Wyer's study involving participants in the publication and in presentations about their research. Here too, it was possible to disseminate the relevant video materials quite widely.

BOX 8.4: A case study of involving participants in the publication and presentation of VRE research

Mary Wyer is a VRE researcher and practising registered nurse. One of her key recommendations from her study of patient involvement in hospital infection prevention and control is for health professionals to consider patients as active partners in preventing health care-associated infections (HAIs). Wyer extends this approach of considering patients as active partners to her own research practice with VRE. Along with Aileen Collier, also a registered nurse, Wyer is one of the first scholars to actively engage patients (rather than only clinical staff) in VRE, both as a co-author and as a co-presenter of VRE results. Wyer and Collier give the title 'co-researcher' to their patient-collaborators (Collier and Wyer, 2016; Wyer, 2017). One of Wyer's patient co-researchers, Gary Armstrong, has co-authored a peer-reviewed publication and several academic conference presentations, and is involved as a consumer member in three different hospital committees as a result of his involvement in Wyer's research. Armstrong's co-research status is more than a name listed among other academic co-authors. As co-author of a VRE article titled 'Should I stay or should I go? Patient understandings of and responses to source-isolation practices', Armstrong helped prepare and review the manuscript, and wrote an epilogue on his experience of having a HAI and being involved in research on HAIs. Wyer requested funding for him to attend and co-present, but this was turned down, so she videoed Armstrong delivering his contribution, and played that video footage to the audience. This footage has since been used for mandatory training by all NSW Health staff (Health Education and Training Institute, personal communication 28 June 2017). Other patient co-researchers in Wyer's study had acquired infection or colonization with multi drug-resistant organisms (MROs). Recognizing that the public dissemination of this potentially stigmatizing condition may present risks (Mozzillo et al., 2010; Rump et al., 2016), but also offer benefits, she stated, 'I negotiated with patient co-researchers which footage or pictures would be used (if any) and whether they wanted their faces blurred. These patients decided that the need for a better understanding of the challenges faced by patients around HAI trumped their desire for anonymity' (Wyer, 2017). Summarizing her experience of collaborating with patients in her work, Wyer states, 'the effect of the strength of our relationships and shared understandings has made us 'more' than we were before' (Wyer, 2017). She continues, '[patient collaborators] have taught me how to conduct respectful and ethical research and have inspired me to have regular, ongoing conversations with the patients I have cared for'. Armstrong's sentiments are similar: 'these conversations, committees and writing opportunities have helped me to better understand infection transmission and prevention, what happened to me, and how I could take better care of my health in the future' (Wyer et al., 2015).

In Mesman's work, the public and identifiable footage portrays a highly skilled and innovative team of professionals taking up VRE to optimize their skilled practices. By contrast, Wyer's footage features patients with a potentially stigmatized condition: a transmissible MRO colonization/infection. And yet, these patients were comfortable with their footage being publicly shown. In general, however, we need to carefully consider our use of footage that depicts particularly sensitive situations or stigmatized illnesses and assume that full confidentiality and anonymity remain our first point of departure (Cox et al., 2014).

As noted earlier, an appropriately ethical stance towards the collection, use and dissemination of visual images is anchored in iterative consent. This includes monitoring and anticipating the many uses and potential futures of visual images. Here, it is important to acknowledge that, were a moving image to be viewed in circumstances outside of our control, it is difficult or impossible to anticipate and manage audiences' responses to the footage. This is particularly the case when the footage fails to be properly framed and contextualized by those directly involved. Indeed, in some cases, participants have regretted sharing their personal information as time went by (Cox et al., 2014).

In a retrospective publication of a larger visual methods project, Wills and colleagues offer particularly sound advice in this regard:

> … the lessons learnt during this study have led some of the authors to approach consent differently in other projects involving visual research methods, asking participants at the end of data collection to more fully consider the consent they wish to give regarding the dissemination of data that identifies a household; only when a researcher or participant knows what data have been gathered can consent be fully discussed.

> *(Wills et al., 2016: 481)*

The issues raised by Mesman's and Wyer's case studies presented above are typical of visual research where there has been an intentional blurring of 'boundaries between the roles of researchers, participants, artists and others' involved' (Cox et al., 2014: 15). As seen, such engagements create opportunities but also complexities that may impact on how the projects' findings are disseminated.

8.7 REPRESENTING AND REPLICATING THE REAL?

As noted in Chapter 1, visuals only capture fragments of what happened in reality, as does language. This point is at the heart of Wills and colleagues' warning that we should not underestimate the extent to which visuals 'downplay' reality. Wills and colleagues in fact regard videoing, editing, cropping, blurring and rendering as essentially 'misrepresenting' the complexity of what is shown. Thus, they ask,

> if ... we choose or rely on particular images or particular kinds of images ... to support what we write about in journal articles or conference presentations, does this misrepresent the complexity of the social practices that we aimed to investigate at the outset? What effect does cropping and blurring – effectively disembodying images from their owners and contexts – have ...?
>
> (Wills et al., 2016: 481)

As already pointed out with reference to Rose's (2016) work, Wills and colleagues qualify images and moving images as no more than 'a version of events coproduced by the filmmaker, photographer and the viewer':

> ... video footage and photographs, whether produced by participants or researchers, are not a taken-for-granted record of everyday life. They are a representation, a version of events coproduced by the filmmaker, photographer and the viewer and subject to interpretation by each of these (as well as other audiences), as with any other source of data. Images also do not become data until layered with interpretation and analysis.
>
> (Wills et al., 2016: 476)

Our desire to include visuals in publications and representations should therefore be mitigated with the acknowledgement that while visuals may broaden readers' and listeners' responses to and insight into our projects, the (moving) images are not capable of transparently conveying what happened. No resource can do this. But what (moving) images do make available is a range of impressions and experiences that text-only and numbers-only studies cannot reproduce. Visuals extend our meaning-making repertoire, and their multi-modal nature (colour, sound, movement and so forth) expands the ways in which we confront and are able to reflect on our living and working circumstances.

In Table 8.2, we summarize the above discussion by formulating a number of critical questions that should be asked when you're intending to publish your VRE project.

Table 8.2 The four guiding principles of VRE: Publishing VRE

Guiding principle	Questions to consider when publishing VRE work
Exnovation	How much context or specificity is needed in the image to meaningfully convey new or impactful knowledge or practice change to wider (non-project) audiences?
	Is a video or photographic image necessary to convey exnovation, or can complex practices and new realizations about that practice be conveyed through texts such as quotations, vignettes or narratives?
Collaboration	Who will store, host and control the availability of images for dissemination?
	Who is involved in the dissemination and publication of images?
	Who is involved in editing or reproducing images and writing text for publication and dissemination?
	Who is involved in interpreting and representing images to diverse or multidisciplinary audiences in presentations or publications (e.g., clinical audience vs social science audience)?
	Who retains the copyright of stored, hosted or disseminated images?
Reflexivity	How is 'giving voice' to participants through visibility and recognizability balanced with confidentiality and anonymity that may involve the silencing of individuals?
	Is there an over-reliance on certain images at the expense of misrepresenting the complexity of healthcare practice or illness experiences?
	Is it necessary to return to participants featured in images to show them images prior to publication in order to obtain further consent?
Care	Whose permissions to you need to seek to disseminate an image?
	How are issues of consent for image dissemination decided with participants?
	Are there opportunities for participants to engage in iterative or processual consent once images have been generated and viewed?
	How is comprehension of 'in perpetuity' tested with participants regarding image dissemination?
	How are issues of participant voice, confidentiality, anonymity, representation and image permanence theorized and actualized in the processes of wider dissemination? Who is invited to become involved in this decision-making process?

8.8 CONCLUSION

This chapter has discussed the issues that arise in relation to the dissemination of VRE studies. Critical issues apply in particular to choices about whether and how to include visuals in publications and presentations. The chapter has sketched out various scenarios where sensitivities arose and how these were overcome. We have listed questions for you to consider in separate tables, reminding you to carefully consider the implications arising from your use of (moving) images.

REFERENCES

Brossard B and Sapin-Leduc A. (2017) Reconnaître et représenter des compétences: le travail relationnel des préposés aux bénéficiaires dans les CHSLD du Québec. *Vie et vieillissement* 14: 20–24.

Carroll K and Mesman J. (2011) Ethnographic context meets ethnographic biography: A challenge for the mores of doing fieldwork. *International Journal of Multiple Research Approaches* 5: 155–168.

Carroll, K and Mesman, J. (2018) Multiple researcher roles in video reflexive ethnography. *Qualitative Health Research* 28, 1145–1156.

Carroll K, Iedema R and Kerridge R. (2008) Reshaping ICU ward round practices using video reflexive ethnography. *Qualitative Health Research* 18: 380–390.

Carroll K, Mesman J, McLeod H, et al. (2018) Seeing what works: Identifying and enhancing successful interprofessional teamwork between pathology and surgery. *Journal of Interprofessional Care.* doi: 10.1080/13561820.2018.1536041.

Carroll K. (2009) Unpredictable predictables: Complexity theory and the construction of order in intensive care. Unpublished PhD Thesis. Sydney: Centre for Health Communication, University of Technology Sydney.

Carroll K. (2015) Representing ethnographic data through the epistolary form. *Qualitative Inquiry* 21: 686–695.

Collier A and Wyer M. (2016) Researching reflexively with patients and families: Two studies using video-reflexive ethnography to collaborate with patients and families in patient safety research. *Qualitative Health Research* 26: 979–993.

Collier A, Sorensen R and Iedema R. (2016) Patients' and families' perspectives of patient safety at the end of life: A video-reflexive ethnography study. *International Journal for Quality in Health Care* 28: 66–73.

Collier A. (2013) Deleuzians of patient safety: A video reflexive ethnography of end-of-life care. Unpublished PhD Thesis. Sydney: Faculty of Arts and Social Sciences, University of Technology.

Cox S, Drew S, Guillemin M, et al. (2014) *Guidelines for Ethical Visual Research Methods*, Melbourne: Visual Research Collaboratory, University of Melbourne.

Dieckmann P, Patterson M, Lahlou S, et al. (2017) Variation and adaptation: Comments on learning from success in simulation training. *Advances in Simulation* 2: 2–21.

Edmondson A. (1999) Psychological safety and learning behavior in work teams. *Administrative Science Quarterly* 44(2): 350–383.

European Union. (2018) General data protection regulation. *Official Journal of the European Union (EU)* OJ L 119, 4.5.2016, p. 1–88

Forsyth R. (2006) *Tricky Technology, Troubled Tribes: A Video Ethnographic Study of the Impact of Information Technology on Health Care Professionals' Practices and Relationships.* PhD Thesis. New South Wales: University of New South Wales.

Forsyth R. (2009) Distance versus dialogue: Modes of engagement of two professional groups participating in a hospital-based video ethnographic study. *International Journal of Multiple Research Approaches* 3: 276–289.

Foster V. (2009) Authentic representation? Using video as counter-hegemony in participatory research with poor working-class women. *International Journal of Multiple Research Approaches* 3: 233–245.

Grant J and Luxford Y. (2009) Video: A decolonizing strategy for intercultural communication in child and family health within ethnographic research international. *Journal of Multiple Research Approaches* 3: 218–232.

Hor S, Hooker C, Iedema R, et al. (2017) Beyond hand hygiene: A qualitative study of the everyday work of preventing cross-contamination on hospital wards. *BMJ Quality & Safety* 26: 552–558.

Hor S, Iedema R and Manias E. (2014) Creating spaces in intensive care for safe communication: A video-reflexive ethnographic study. *BMJ Quality & Safety* 23: 1007–1013.

Hor S and Iedema R. (2015) In: Collyer, F. (ed.) Bruno Latour: From acting at a distance towards matters of concern in patient safety. In: *The Palgrave Handbook of Social Theory in Health, Illness and Medicine.* Pallgrave Macmillan, Basingstoke, 660–674.

Iedema R. (2011) Creating safety by strengthening clinicians' capacity for reflexivity. *BMJ Quality and Safety* 20: S83–S86.

Iedema R and Bezemer J. (under review) Researching health care complexity: Towards transformative engagement. *BMC Medicine.*

Iedema R and Carroll K. (2015) Research as affect-sphere: Towards spherogenics. *Emotion Review* 7: 1–7.

Iedema R, Ball C, Daly B, et al. (2012) Design and trial of a new ambulance-to-emergency department handover protocol: 'IMIST-AMBO'. *BMJ Quality & Safety* 21: 627–633.

Iedema R, Long D and Carroll K. (2010) Corridor communication, spatial design and patient safety: Enacting and managing complexities. In: Van Marrewijk A and Yanow D (eds) *Space, Meaning and Organisation.* Cheltenham: Edward Elgar, 41–57.

Iedema R, Long D, Forsyth R, et al. (2006) Visibilizing clinical work: Video ethnography in the contemporary hospital. *Health Sociology Review* 15: 156–168.

Iedema R, Merrick E, Rajbhandari D, et al. (2009) Viewing the taken-for-granted from under a different aspect: A video-based method in pursuit of patient safety. *International Journal for Multiple Research Approaches* 3: 290–301.

Iedema R, Mesman J and Carroll K. (2013) *Visualising Health Care Practice Improvement: Innovation from Within.* London: Radcliffe.

Lammer C. (2009) Empathograhies: Using body art related video approaches in the environment of an Australian teaching hospital. *International Journal of Multiple Research Approaches* 3: 264–275.

Leap N, Sandall J, Grant J, et al. (2009) Using video in the development and field-testing of a learning package for maternity staff: Supporting women for normal childbirth. *International Journal of Multiple Research Approaches* 3: 302–320.

Lenne B. (2018) The autism diagnostic encounter in action: Using video reflexive ethnography to explore the assessment of autism in the clinical trial. Unpublished PhD Thesis. Sydney: University of Sydney.

Mannay D. (2016) *Visual, Narrative and Creative Research Methods: Application, Reflection and Ethics.* Abingdon, Oxon: Routledge.

McLeod H. (2017) Respect and shared decision making in the clinical encounter: A video-reflexive ethnography. PhD Thesis. University of Minnesota.

Mesman J. (2011) Resources of strength: An exnovation of hidden competences to preserve patient safety. In: Rowley E and Waring J (eds) *A Sociocultural Perspective on Patient Safety.* Farnham: Ashgate, 71–92.

Mesman J. (2015) Boundary spanning engagement on the neonatal ward: Reflections on a collaborative entanglement between clinicians and a researcher. In: Penders B, Vermeulen N and Parker J (eds) *Collaboration across Health Research and Medical Care.* Farnham: Ashgate, 171–194.

Mozzillo KL, Ortiz N and Miller LG. (2010) Patients with meticillin-resistant Staphylococcus aureus infection: Twenty-first century lepers. *Journal of Hospital Infection* 75: 132–134.

Rose G. (2016) *Visual Methodologies: An Introduction to Researching with Visual Materials.* Los Angeles, CA: Sage.

Rump B, De Boer MG, Reis R, et al. (2016) Signs of stigma and poor mental health among carriers of methicillin-resistant staphylococcus aureus. *Open Forum Infectious Diseases* suppl–1, Oxford University Press, S1.

Sormani P, Alac M, Bovet A, et al. (2017) Ethnomethodology, video analysis, and STS. In: Felt U, Fouché R, Miller C, et al. (eds) *The Handbook of Science and Technology Studies,* 4th edition. Cambridge, MA: The MIT Press.

Stone PW, Pogorzelska-Maziarz M, Reagan J, et al. (2015) Impact of laws aimed at healthcare-associated infection reduction: A qualitative study. *BMJ Quality & Safety* 24: 637–644.

Van Helmond I, Korstjens I, Mesman J, et al. (2015) What makes for good collaboration and communication in maternity care? A scoping study. *International Journal of Childbirth* 5: 210–223.

Wills W, Dickinson A, Meah A, et al. (2016) Reflections on the use of visual methods in a qualitative study of domestic kitchen practices. *Sociology* 50: 470–485.

Wyer M. (2017) Integrating patients' experiences, understandings and enactments of infection prevention and control into clinicians' everyday care: A video-reflexive ethnographic exploratory intervention. PhD Thesis. University of Tasmania, Hobart, Australia.

Wyer M, Iedema R, Jorm C, et al. (2015) Should I stay or should I go? Patient understandings of and responses to source-isolation practices. *Patient Experience Journal* 2: 60–68.

9

Tying the principal strands of the book together

9.1 INTRODUCTION

This chapter concludes our book. This last chapter will not summarize what has come before. Instead, we will take the opportunity to expand some of the more theoretical issues and questions raised in our Introduction and Chapter 1, and flesh out the main defining characteristics of the thinking that underpin video-reflexive ethnography (VRE).

Section 9.2 delves more deeply into the links between VRE and complexity theory. This section connects to the next one, which addresses the reasons for VRE to prioritize learning and asking over knowing and stating. We conclude the chapter with a brief consideration of the role of the camera in learning about complexity.

9.2 VRE AND COMPLEXITY THEORY

As we stated in previous chapters, VRE wants to tackle health care where it is at its most complex. Care is that domain of interactions where healthcare professionals, patients and families work out diagnoses, treatments, tests, as well as palliative and all kinds of other clinical and care-management activities. This care unfolds in time and space, in the present, or in the 'here-and-now'. Put differently, we can walk into a health service and observe care as it takes place in all its manifestations. This may involve nurses speaking with patients while doctors are doing a ward round and ward managers are busy liaising with colleagues on the phone. Cleaners push trolleys with bins and brushes, while others move patients in wheel chairs. If asked, we could produce a description of such care by detailing what it looks like now, in the present, or the here and now.

We defined this here-and-now care as the zone of maximum complexity. Our justification for characterizing care in this way is that the here-and-now acts as the 'collection point' for several 'runaway' developments. Think of the increasingly younger and increasingly older patients presenting with rising numbers of diseases or multi-morbidities (Hughes et al., 2013). Patients over the age of 60 tend to have at least three diseases (Yu et al., 2016). Looking after these patients with mounting levels of multi-morbidity, clinicians have to oversee and manage more and more treatments, drugs, technologies, specialties and tests (Brown and Webster, 2004).

Making matters more complex still, science, and the medical and clinical sciences in particular, display runaway characteristics: on top of more and more trials being conducted around the world, there is also more knowledge that is disputed and evidence that is contradicted, thus producing more uncertainty (Arbesman, 2012). A recent study found 40% of trials examined have had their findings overturned (Prasad et al., 2013). These knowledge uncertainties are compounded by 'people churn' in health care: staff and patients are subject to increasing mobility and migration. Team relationships and memberships are unstable (West and Lyubovnikova, 2012). Services are more frequently being redesigned and restructured (Braithwaite et al., 2007), and bureaucratic and regulatory pressures in the form of reporting, monitoring, policy updates, accreditation and the like are intensifying (Greenhalgh, 2012). Thanks to technological advances resulting in more treatment options and care decisions for patients, the ethical tensions in health care are exacerbating (Agledahl et al., 2011), and the resources available to cope with these changes are shrinking. Collectively, these factors converge upon the here-and-now activities of doctors, nurses, allied health staff and managers, and upon the here-and-now care received by patients.

And yet, this complexity of how here-and-now care unfolds amidst these pressures and developments is rarely allowed to come to the fore. At times they may surface when ethnographers publish their in-depth findings, or when inquiries delve into the origins and details of a healthcare scandal (Kennedy, 2001; Francis, 2013). Unhelpfully, health research has tended to privilege sophisticated, specialized and 'distanced' ways of converting care realities into data. Prominent here are medical record analyses (Classen et al., 2011) and statistical process control analyses (Carey and Lloyd, 2001), to name but some approaches that are available to practice improvement researchers and clinicians (Shekelle et al., 2013). For their part, and admittedly, ethnography and real-time observations of the unfolding of care are also becoming more accepted in healthcare improvement research (Lingard et al., 2006).

Indeed, at present there are calls for closer attention to be paid to the work 'as done' (Hollnagel, 2015). The reasoning here is that work as it is done harbours what Hollnagel and colleagues refer to as unmapped reservoirs of resilience (Braithwaite et al., 2015). We are advised that, instead of viewing health care as deficient and focus on what goes wrong, we should appreciate the 'great deal of success in things going right' (Braithwaite et al., 2015: 420). Thus, we are told that

> clinicians successfully adjust what they do to match the conditions [and] front-line staff facilitate and manage their work flexibly and safely.
>
> (Braithwaite et al., 2015: 419)

In emphasizing front-line clinicians' resilience, these commentators move the pendulum from our focus on safety incidents and practice improvement, towards greater appreciation of what clinicians do. This would be a significant step forward, were these proposals to be accompanied by methodological innovations. Their reliance on conventional methods means these proposals are ultimately unable to offer additional insight into the complexity of care.

As VRE studies have demonstrated, front-line clinicians themselves neither overestimate their own successes and resilience, nor do they regard their own practices as incident-ridden and deficient. On the contrary, reviewing their work on video highlights for them the immense complexity and richness of their own care practices. In earlier chapters we described this impact of video on participants by invoking the term 'hologram', in so far that reviewing video footage generally reveals practice to harbour all kinds of historical, contextual, habitual, systemic, and consequential dimensions as well meliorative opportunities. Video footage foregrounds that which is commonly taken for granted, and which most people have learned to ignore.

For those embroiled in everyday care practice, witnessing how care unfolds in the 'here and now' has untold merit. As explained and demonstrated in previous chapters, people are enabled to appreciate the complexity of what they do, and grasp how they can act on that complexity. This is because VRE does not erase complexity from view, and instead puts participants in the position of needing to comprehend and address that complexity themselves.

If healthcare improvement and research have to date insisted on converting real-time care into abstractions (numerical data), ethnography and observation have as their aim to expand our understanding of the details and logics of care. These are not just different ways of information gathering, or even different routes to complementary kinds of information. Some methods – VRE included – foreground (aside from other things) the experiential and emotional dimensions of care. Experiencing care as it unfolds opens us up to more than information: the experience moves us, it affects us. We speak about experience here to acknowledge that life can be complex and difficult. We can take in the beauty of a well-functioning and highly complicated machine, but we tend to reserve the term 'experience' for events that harbour complexity, and which therefore affect us emotionally. Care is more than a complicated machine whose parts we can perfect off-site. Care is also an experience, for both clinicians and patients.

Given the emotional intensity that is often associated with illness and illness treatment, it is a little surprising that healthcare improvement commonly anchors progress to methodological procedures and scientific programmes where feelings are relegated to a marginal role, if any. In such work, formal knowledge, data collection and analysis, scientific evidence, bureaucratic directives and interpersonal techniques are seen to be adequate and sufficient for understanding complexity and occasioning change. While practice improvement and health professional education now target 'non-technical skills' (Flin, 2017), and implementation science acknowledges the critical roles of relationships and personal habits in change (Nilsen et al., 2012), these shifts have as yet limited effect when it comes to appointing *methods* for studying and evoking these relational and interpersonal phenomena. Complexity science may now inform these various endeavours, but its privileging of abstract concepts and principles will limit if not in fact obstruct engagement with experienced complexity, and with the emotionality that permeates these experiences.

Let's put this point in somewhat different terms, because it is crucial to the premises of this book, and to our ability to reshape healthcare improvement. In essence, we argue that complexity as such demands not only more attention but also a different kind of attention than we are currently granting it (Wilden, 1980). We currently still prioritize the need for *a priori* 'understanding' of complexity phenomena over practical opportunities to engage with complexity as it manifests itself *in situ* to those embroiled in that complexity. But what does it mean to 'understand' complex phenomena? Does it mean that we can actually predict how such phenomena will play out in real time? Or does it mean that we are prepared for phenomena to radically change course, and that we are humble with regard to the understandings and knowledge that we have gathered to date?

To tackle these questions, let's briefly rehearse the premise of complexity as it was introduced into scientific thinking by Ilya Prigogine. Prigogine (1917–2003) was a physical chemist whose exposition on 'dissipative structures' and self-organizing, non-linear systems won him the Nobel Prize (Prigogine and Stengers, 1984). Prigogine and Stengers' view of nature, physics and chemistry led them to posit that, for them, 'stability and simplicity are exceptions' (Prigogine and Stengers, 1984: 216).

Not much later, Prigogine (1996) published his book titled *The End of Certainty*. In this book, he sets out his more recent views on complexity. His theory sought to highlight the shifting relationship between stability and instability. Phenomena are or become complex when their stability is challenged by emergent (unpredictable) events. Imagine an intensive care unit where in one afternoon four patients are discovered to have infectious diseases and therefore need to be moved into isolation rooms that may be already occupied. Staff have to work hard to re-establish order. This requires resilience (Woods, 2006). But no amount of resilience may be enough when complexity turns into chaos, or the sense that things are well out of control. Chaos means there is a complete lack of stability and predictability. Imagine the following: The number of patients that are infected and in need of being moved balloons. Clinicians' tasks, decisions and reasoning are beginning to cut across one another in confusing ways. For junior clinicians on duty, risk levels rise exponentially.

Hospital-acquired infection investigations have done much to enable us to understand how patients become infected, what measures contribute most effectively to limiting cross-infection, how staff can be persuaded to wash their hands more frequently and thoroughly and how reducing the use of antibiotics contributes to limiting anti-microbial resistance (O'Neil, 2014). These are all important angles on the problem. But they only serve to emphasize those dimensions of care that can be mechanized.

Professionals and patients deal with infection in the here and now. Even if we may find it difficult to think about infection in this way due to its 'invisibility', infection occurs as specific – albeit *complex* – event, action and experience.

Hence, infection registers not just as lesions on patients' bodies but also in orga-nized attempts at its prevention (hand-washing, gloving, gowning, ward decon-tamination, strain typing) and in people's decisions, assumptions and questions about its manifestation and risk (Iedema et al., 2018). Along the lines of Latour's thought exercise applied to face-to-face interaction discussed in Chapter 1, infection control practice might therefore also be traced across time and space as follows:

> We say, without giving the matter too much thought, that we engage in infection control. Indeed we do, but the infection con-trol rules we are following come from elsewhere and were drafted some time ago; the strategies we apply may not have been articu-lated for this specific occasion; the spaces where we practice infec-tion control were designed for purposes and by designers whose rationales may not fully align with the imperatives of infection control but which continue to make themselves felt. The very per-son (or people) we are targeting with our infection control mea-sures bring(s) a history of life experiences and social interactions that goes far beyond our here-and-now relationship. If we were to attempt to draw a spatio-temporal map of what plays a role in our infection control activity, and draw up a comprehensive list of infection risks, we would not sketch out a well-demarcated frame, but a constantly shifting, convoluted multiplicity of highly diverse infection sources, routes, and effects.

> *(adapted from and with apologies to Bruno Latour!)*

Professionals and patients are very well placed to scrutinize and illuminate the local transmission of infectious agents – or at least, to consider the behaviours that may act as vehicles for their transmission (Iedema et al., 2015). We thus sug-gest that paying attention to *in situ* behaviour in areas with high cross-infection risk may throw new light on such risk and on infection routes (Iedema et al., 2015). Those with familiarity of the *in situ* behaviour shown in the video footage may appreciate the logic of what is unfolding, and understand its *ecology*. This is what makes participants so central to VRE: their embeddedness in everyday care practices makes them best placed for not just spotting where stability risks top-pling over into instability; their embeddedness also makes them best placed for identifying rescue and improvement opportunities.

This brings us back to a point we made in Chapter 1, where we advocated for engaging with complexity *in situ* as the means *par excellence* for strengthening our ability to discern its 'structures'. The strategy articulated there was to immerse ourselves in the complexities of everyday care (by videoing them and replaying them), and therefore move 'from the complex to *the structures of complexity*' (Wilden, 1987: 314). This strategy invests faith in local actors' ability to discern 'the structures of complexity' amidst the complex circumstances they inhabit.

With this, the conception that complexity necessarily harbours risk and needs to be tamed and subjected to simplification (knowledge, standardization) may be somewhat revised. Consider that simplicity and linearity don't require much of our attention and afford increasingly automatized responses. Simplicity attenuates attention. It follows that complexity by contrast intensifies our attention and as such is a requisite aspect of our being in the world. Complexity vitalizes, it draws our interest, it maintains our attention and it demands action and intervention (even if that comes down to help-seeking). Complexity may be challenging, but it both obliges and enables us to assert our agency, our creativity and our personal and professional relevance. Complexity makes us realize our unique contribution to progressing care and keeping it safe.

9.3 VRE AND THE PRIMACY OF LEARNING

Given that the complexities just described manifest in the here and now, and given that professionals' and patients' moment-to-moment activities are inevitably instrumental in some way or another to in-hospital cross-infection, professionals and patients are central to working out how infection risks and complexities may be addressed and prevented. Their centrality derives not merely from the fact that, as the 'last pair of hands', for them containing infection risk is a duty, but also from the fact that they may be able to strengthen their own infection control intelligence through scrutinizing and reshaping the habits that undergird their infection control.

In contrast to a human factors' view which tends to emphasize humans' limitations (Zinck-Pedersen, 2018), we prefer to see individuals in a more variegated way. People are steeped in taken-as-given habits that may have lost their currency, relevance and intelligence, but people are also and nevertheless the prime locus of agency and learning. After all, they are the 'means' through which general guidelines, abstract knowledge, formal evidence, off-the-shelf solutions, technological resources, cultural proclivities, practical experiences, local opportunities and emergent events become integrated into actual and yet-to-unfold ways of being and doing. Their learning and their agency are therefore central to how we apprehend complexity and how we act amidst complexity.

This is the reason that VRE brings individuals' learning and agency to the fore. Yeats is claimed to have said that learning is not about filling buckets but about lighting fires. Yeats' dictum reappears in a somewhat more scholarly form in Gert Biesta's distinction between knowing as appropriating (regarding the world as at my disposal) and learning as becoming more caring and receptive towards 'what is'.

> When we think of knowing as reception the world does not 'appear' as an object that is at our disposal but rather as 'something' that comes to us. Knowing then is not an act of mastery or control – our 'attitude' to the world, natural and social, is not technological – but can perhaps better be described as a process of listening to the world, of having a concern for the world, of caring for the world.
>
> *(Biesta, 2015: 238/239)*

Biesta's (2015: 238) view tackles head-on the problem that defines conventional science, namely that 'through my act of [scientific] knowing I try to master the world':

> This [conventional aim] means that [I wrongly assume that] in a very fundamental sense my existence 'occurs' before the existence of the world: I assume that I am there first in order then to start making sense of the world. It also means that I assume that the world exists *for* me, that is, that the world is in some way at my disposal as an object for me to make sense of and construct knowledge about.
>
> *(Biesta, 2015: 238)*

Biesta questions our 'technical engagement with the world' because it presupposes that we are in control. This is more than evident from how we study and act on the world, presupposing 'a primacy of method, of procedure, of research methods over objects [investigated]' (Sloterdijk, 1983: 359). Sloterdijk (1983: 359/360) regards scientific 'rigour', so prominent an ideal in healthcare research and improvement circles, as being 'procured at the cost of a methodological constriction or standardization of what the subject [researcher, clinician] is allowed or not allowed to "know"'.

VRE distinguishes itself from these kinds of 'technical engagement with the world'. Previous chapters have emphasized that VRE is not methodologically constricted beyond an emphasis on exnovation, the reliance on participation by practitioners and patients, the use of footage as attention-focusing resource to engender reflexivity as deliberative change dynamic and an ethic of care for participants. VRE creates footage of naturally occurring practices, and such footage need not be subjected to predetermined kinds of analysis (privileging neither fixed views on clinical expertise nor prefigured measurements). Here, footage is shown merely to elicit discussions about complex aspects of everyday work. In this way, VRE inspires participants to apprehend and learn about clinical, practical and systems complexities, since VRE 'approaches [these complexities] … not as master researcher … but as neighbour, friend, as someone who has been "drawn in"' (Sloterdijk, 1983: 359/360).

'Being drawn in' defines VRE's research and improvement strategy (Iedema and Carroll, 2015). Based on this, VRE is methodologically, procedurally and thematically agnostic. That is, interviews, shadowing, focus groups, reflexive feedback, *ad hoc* discussions are all part and parcel of furthering VRE relationships, deliberations, learning and change. Clinical handover, infection control, end of life, autism, respect in care, breast milk use in neonatal intensive care units, patients' experiences and more are all open to VRE intervention. Its overarching aim is learning; not learning as knowing more, but learning as 'opening up to'. Such learning respects the complexity of care as it unfolds, as well as the experiences of those involved and the logic of what is possible and necessary.

Biesta's 'opening up to the world' is not dissimilar to VRE's reflexive process. By involving front-line professionals and patients in addressing local problems, we seek to enhance these people's ability to act, or their *agency*. Their transformation into becoming more effective actors is not achieved through being given more relevant or "truer" information. On the contrary, it is achieved on the strength of their being affected by what they see and by what they and others say about it. This, in turn, affects their power to act because they have opened up to (how they negotiate) *in situ* circumstances, challenges and complexities. Being affected by the VRE process thus means opening up to how everyday care unfolds, since 'the greater our power to be affected ... the greater our power to act' (Hardt, 2007: x).

9.4 VRE'S FOCUS ON 'THE HERE-AND-NOW'

The section above helps explain another critical point: why VRE targets the here and now. We just saw that enhancing people's power to act means enhancing their power to be affected. People are affected by what happens in the here-and-now: their experience of what happens to them and others around them. Particularly, complex experiences affect people, as they cannot but negotiate a unique path through such experiences. This last point raises the possibility that complexity is at the heart of human experience per se, as it vitalizes people's connections, relevance and agency. Equally, and while it defines the aims and objectives of complexity scientific endeavours in health care, 'taming' complexity is not the only route to improvement and safety. Embracing and harnessing complexity to bolster people's engagement, agency and inventiveness may in fact be more relevant to 21st-century healthcare circumstances, and more appropriate to contemporary healthcare processes and relationships.

Research approaches that set store by everyday experiences tend to satisfy themselves with collecting people's memories and opinions in the form of 'narratives' (Greenhalgh et al., 2005). Processed as narratives however, these experiences have already been reshaped to suit forms and formats that background the intense complexity of the events themselves. Experiences are no longer replayed in real time, but now conform to narrative time. In contrast to this, VRE sets store by retrieving everyday experiences in as unprocessed a form and format as possible: as visual footage capturing events in real time.

As we described in our 2008 article (Carroll et al., 2008), reviewing experiences as video footage helps people gain some distance from what happened, while at the same time bringing these experiences closer. As the footage grants us a novel perspective on what is familiar ('footage distances') what happened can look strange. At the same time, the footage showing what happened creates an intense sense of recognition, since it is we (or colleagues) who are on show. This dual movement enables participants to see themselves and others 'from under a different aspect' (Wittgenstein, 1953; Iedema et al., 2009), and this opens up what Massumi refers to as a 'space of transformation' (Massumi, 2002: 52). Reviewing footage of *in situ* practice connects people to experiences in new ways: doing so affords them new ways of seeing, new ways of experiencing and new ways of acting.

For these reasons, VRE differs from implementation scientific endeavours, whose common aim is to account for a generalizable logic of complexity that governs all local contexts (May et al., 2016). For implementation science as for healthcare practice improvement generally, the research-cum-improvement trajectory *par excellence* is as identified above: 'proceeding from the "simple" to the "complex" (as 17th century "empiricists" and ideologists like John Locke (1632–1704) thought we should and could)' (Wilden, 1987: 314). The thinking undergirding this trajectory is not 'complexity thinking'. This is because its roots reach deep into 'simplicity thinking' that effectively treats 'the system… as an object, and moreover as an object to be viewed or even "controlled" from an imaginary "outside"' (Wilden, 1980: xxxviii).

VRE renders engaging with complex circumstances conditional neither on 'understanding the dimensions of complexity' nor on the deployment of conventional data gathering methods that objectify the aspects of complex circumstances. Instead of giving primacy to generalization and simplification, VRE gives primacy to complexity and specificity by positing that

1. Local people play a critical role in the process of resolving complex *in situ* problems.
2. Local people's interest, concern and confidence to address and act amidst complexity may be sparked by showing them video footage of *in situ* practice.
3. By reviewing footage of *in situ* complexities, people can connect in novel ways to otherwise taken-for-granted and non-questioned events and experiences.
4. People's sense of agency, relevance and inventiveness are strengthened through their experiences and deliberations about those experiences being granted a generative role in safety and improvement.

Now, the prominence for VRE of the 'here and now' is justified as follows: Leaving modelling and formal analyses to other endeavours, VRE regards complexity as needing to be tackled there where (and when) it manifests itself in people's lives, such that those people's own ability to act and intervene in the here-and-now complexity is enhanced. In taking this view, VRE aligns itself with the views of other complexity theorists:

> … the way change happens and the way the future emerges is dependent on the detailed and particular events and patterns of relationships and particular features in the local situation.
>
> *(Boulton et al., 2015: 8)*

Boulton and colleagues further note that

> … the only reliable way to investigate the way things are, and certainly the way things change, is through paying attention to the local detail.
>
> *(Boulton et al., 2015: 10)*

Supporting this focus on the 'here and now', in a recent book on patient safety, Zinck Pedersen (2018: 216) identifies 'the clinical situation' as a critical starting point for healthcare improvement research. In our earlier book (Iedema et al., 2013), we identified 'the (clinical) work' as it unfolds in real time as the critical focus of our research. Accordingly, VRE captures and portrays how care unfolds from moment to moment, without privileging critical moments (emergencies, resuscitations, surgical procedures) at the expense of more mundane ones on the view that the latter afford as much, if not more, learning.

9.5 THE SIGNIFICANCE OF THE CAMERA AND OF VISION

If the focus of healthcare research and improvement should include the here-and-now, then the question becomes: How do we grant the 'here and now' a role in how we do research and learning? Remember that the principal research question for VRE is not 'How can we explain and model complexity?', since answers to this question may be out of date by the time they are formulated, they may be out of sync with the experiences and interests of local actors and they may be unrepresentative of reality by the time they are applied to specific situations. Instead, VRE posits the principal research question as being: 'How can we all (researchers, research participants) become better at recognizing and acting amidst complex situations?'. This latter question implies another: How do we best engage complexity?

For the most part, language has been the medium *par excellence* through which the questions, analyses, findings and recommendations of healthcare research have been communicated. Yet in this day and age, we make use of vision much more than in the past. Its application in healthcare research remains limited however to cultural studies and artistic endeavours (Pink, 2007), with some exceptions (Mackenzie and Xiao, 2003; Broekhuis and Veldkamp, 2007). The potential or 'affordance' of vision for impacting on health care therefore remains as yet under-appreciated (Iedema et al., 2009). This is all the more surprising given the extensive commentaries about the effects of vision on how we see and experience the world (Deleuze, 1986; Massumi, 2002). As did the advent of print several hundred years ago (Ong, 1992), vision alters our consciousness of things and of ourselves. Specifically, viewing ourselves in footage enables us to enter into a 'space of transformation' where we come to apprehend ourselves as others do, creating movement for us and in us.

This movement, in turn, enables us to intervene in our own habits. Earlier we cited Dewey's work in which he explains that habits are humans' primary entry point into the world. We view the world through our habits, or, as Dewey writes, 'Concrete habits do all the perceiving, recognizing, imagining, recalling, judging, conceiving and reasoning that is done' (Dewey, 1922: 124). As habits however, they tend to be taken as given, and we need distance from them to 'unlock them': 'We cannot unlock our own habits and habituations without at once distancing ourselves from them... [and taking ourselves beyond them]' (Sloterdijk, 2009: 300). This is how we phrased this thinking in our earlier work:

> We feel implicated in video footage because it confronts us with an entirely new perspective from which to apprehend who we are, what we say and what we do. This is not purely about knowing or 'seeing' – it is about experiencing. Its intense effect is due to the

moving image's special qualities. It differs radically from the spoken phrase or the still photo, as Massumi explained in his book *Parables for the Virtual* (2002). The moving image transforms, he said, because it alters our perception and therefore our sense of existence. That is precisely what it does every time we train the camera on ordinary processes in care, and when we display the resulting footage to stakeholders in that care. Because it comes as a series of moving images, video unfolds the performance of care in all its dynamic complexity. It bares who we are and what we do in a way that is neither excessively confronting (as verbal feedback from a colleague might be), nor too forgiving (like, say, a flattering photo). This is because footage reveals that we are deeply connected to others and to ongoing events.

(Iedema et al., 2013: ix)

A final point to make about the camera is that the footage it produces does not merely reflect or mirror events and behaviours. On the contrary, the process of viewing footage is productive, as it creates a new energy for dealing with our taken-for-granted habits, or 'fidelities previously blind' (Dewey, 1922: 55). Indeed, for Dewey, observation

... is not however a mere idle mirroring of pre-existent acts. It is an additional event having its own career. It sets up a heightened emotional appreciation and provides a new motive for fidelities previously blind. It sets up an attitude of criticism, of inquiry, and makes men [sic] sensitive to the brutalities and extravagances of customs.

(Dewey, 1922: 55)

This is the dynamic that drives VRE: people becoming emotionally implicated in and critically attuned to what they see. This dynamic alerts them to 'fidelities [here: habits and customs] previously blind' and renders them 'sensitive to the extravagances of [their habits and] customs'. This reflection on our own 'extravagances of habit' is critical because

The ordinary process of habit formation can no longer be trusted for adjusting to new conditions because it is so slow, unsystematic and uncertain... Given the rapid rate of contemporary change, even if we are lucky enough to develop a good habit unreflectively, it could easily be rendered obsolete by the time it is successfully achieved... We thus need a systematic method for the intelligent reconstruction of habit.

(Shusterman, 2008: 93)

Through seeing themselves implicated and entangled in socially constituted and socially unfolding activity in the footage, professionals and patients come to realize that their actions are not simply motivated by personal reasoning and decision-making. Instead, they realize their actions are largely shaped by habits and customs, by the atmosphere at and conditions of work, by relationships and by others' routines, reasonings and activities (over and above more personal attributes and contributions). Video footage bears these social and systemic dimensions out quite vividly: people are enabled to see themselves as members of communities of practice and as people who inhabit, perform and are steered by practices that have a (historical, contextual, systemic, habituated) logic of their own. While accustomed to construe themselves as thinking individuals, participants witnessing footage come to realize that events are multi-layered, and that their actions harbour a *performed systematicity*.

As individuals, we feel we have responsibility for perpetuating our work practices and their logic, most often because they buttress relationships, cultures, organizations, services and therefore our sense of appropriateness and legitimacy. Video reflexivity alters our grip on ourselves and on our practices, as it enables us to discern previously unappreciated social roots of action and previously unacknowledged cultural logics driving our habits. In alerting us to these things, the footage generates *impulse*. That is, footage represents 'a novel factor in the surroundings [and thereby] releases some impulse which tends to initiate a different and incompatible activity' (Dewey, 1922: 179). Impulse, in Dewey's thinking, is affect or emotion. Without emotion, we may not be able to connect to our experiences or affect our habits. Change may therefore be an illusion if we think it can be achieved in technical, formal and general ways, without engaging us experientially, emotionally, locally and personally.

9.6 CONCLUSION

This section concludes our book. We have attempted to provide everything from a theoretical background to practical tips and philosophical legitimation. Your task will be to realize VRE in ways that make sense to your chosen sites and enthusiastic collaborators. In the end, VRE is no more than the totality of endeavours and outcomes produced by researchers and clinicians interested in engaging with everyday complexity for the purpose of learning and improving care. In tandem with other efforts and approaches, VRE can offer special impetus and elicit unusual levels of energy among those struggling with systems, practices and relationships. One day, the misconception that acting locally has no relevance for the healthcare system as a whole will be revealed for what it is: a ruse distracting us from where care begins and ends, the here and now.

REFERENCES

Agledahl KM, Førde R, and Wifstad A. (2011) Choice is not the issue. The misrepresentation of healthcare in bioethical discourse. *Journal of Medical Ethics* 37: 212–215.

Arbesman S. (2012) *The Half-Life of Facts: Why Everything We Know Has an Expiration Date.* New York: Penguin.

Biesta G. (2015) Freeing teaching from learning: Opening up existential possibilities in educational relationships. *Studies in Philosophy and Education* 34: 229–243.

Boulton J, Allen P, and Bowman C. (2015) *Embracing Complexity: Strategic Perspectives for an Age of Turbulence.* Oxford: Oxford University Press.

Braithwaite J, Wears RL, and Hollnagel E. (2015) Resilient health care: Turning patient safety on its head. *International Journal for Quality in Health Care* 27: 418–420.

Braithwaite J, Westbrook M, Hindle D, et al. (2007) Hospital sector organisational restructuring: Evidence of its futility. In: Ferlie E, Hyde P and McKee L (eds) *Organizing and Reorganizing-Power and Change in Health Care Organizations.* Basingstoke: Palgrave, 33–45.

Broekhuis M and Veldkamp C. (2007) The usefulness and feasibility of a reflexivity method to improve clinical handover. *Journal of Evaluation in Clinical Practice* 13: 109–115.

Brown N and Webster A. (2004) *New Medical Technologies and Society: Reordering Life.* Cambridge: Polity Press.

Carey RG and Lloyd RC. (2001) *Measuring Quality Improvement in Health Care: A Guide to Statistical Process Control Applications.* Milwaukee, WI: American Society for Quality Press.

Carroll K, Iedema R, and Kerridge R. (2008) Reshaping ICU ward round practices using video reflexive ethnography. *Qualitative Health Research* 18: 380–390.

Classen D, Resar RK, Griffin F, et al. (2011) 'Global Trigger Tool' shows that adverse events may be ten times greater than previously measured. *Health Affairs* 4: 581–589.

Deleuze G. (1986) *Cinema 1: The Movement Image.* Minneapolis: University of Minnesota Press.

Dewey J. (1922) *Human Nature and Conduct: An Introduction to Social Psychology.* New York: H. Holt & Company.

Flin R. (2017) Enhancing safety performance: Non-technical skills and a modicum of chronic unease. In: Bieder C, Gilbert C and Laroche H (eds) *Beyond Safety Training: Embedding Safety in Professional Skills.* Cham: Springer, 45–58.

Francis R. (2013) *Report of the Mid Staffordshire NHS Foundation Trust Public Inquiry.* London: The Stationery Office.

Greenhalgh T. (2012) Why do we always end up here? Evidence-based medicine's conceptual cul-de-sacs and some off-road alternative routes. *Journal of Primary Health Care* 4: 92–97.

Greenhalgh T, Russell J and Swinglehurst D. (2005) Narrative methods in quality improvement research. *Quality and Safety in Health Care* 14: 443–449.

Hardt M. (2007) Foreword: What affects are good for. In: Ticineto-Clough P and Halley J (eds) *The Affective Turn: Theorizing the Social.* Durham, NC: Duke University Press, ix–xiii.

Hollnagel E. (2015) Why Is work-as-imagined different from work-as-done? In: Wears RL, Hollnagel E and Braithwaite J (eds) *Resilient Health Care: The Resilience of Everyday Clinical Work*. Farnham: Ashgate, 249–264.

Hughes L, McMurdo M, and Guthrie B. (2013) Guidelines for people not for diseases: The challenges of applying UK clinical guidelines to people with multimorbidity. *Age & Ageing* 42: 62–69.

Iedema R and Carroll K. (2015) Research as affect-sphere: Towards spherogenics. *Emotion Review* 7: 1–7.

Iedema R, Hor S, Wyer M, et al. (2015) An innovative approach to strengthening health professionals' infection control and limiting hospital acquired infection: Video-reflexive ethnography. *BMJ Innovation* 1: 157–162: doi:10.1136/bmjinnov-2014–000032.

Iedema R, Jorm C, Hooker C, et al. (2018) To follow a rule? On frontline clinicians' understandings and embodiments of hospital-acquired infection prevention and control rules. *Health*. doi:10.1177/1363459318785677.

Iedema R, Merrick E, Rajbhandari D, et al. (2009) Viewing the taken-for-granted from under a different aspect: A video-based method in pursuit of patient safety. *International Journal for Multiple Research Approaches* 3: 290–301.

Iedema R, Mesman J, and Carroll K. (2013) *Visualising Health Care Practice Improvement: Innovation from Within*. London: Radcliffe.

Kennedy I. (2001) *The Bristol Royal Infirmary Inquiry*. London: Department of Health.

Lingard L, Whyte S, Espin S, et al. (2006) Towards safer interprofessional communication: Constructing a model of "utility" from preoperative team briefings. *Journal of Interprofessional Care* 20: 471–483.

Mackenzie CF and Xiao Y. (2003) Video techniques and data compared with observation in emergency trauma care. *Journal of Quality and Safety in Health Care* 12 (Suppl II): ii51–ii57.

Massumi B. (2002) *Parables for the Virtual: Movement, Affect, Sensation*. Durham, NC: Duke University Press.

May C, Johnson M, and Finch T. (2016) Implementation, context and complexity. *Implementation Science* 11: 1–12.

Nilsen P, Roback K, Brostrom A, et al. (2012) Creatures of habit: Accounting for the role of habit in implementation research on clinical behaviour change. *Implementation Science* 7: 53. www.implementationscience.com/content/7/1/53

O'Neil J. (2014) *Antimicrobial Resistance: Tackling a Crisis for the Health and Wealth of Nations – The Review on Antimicrobial Resistance*. London: HM Government & Welcome Trust.

Ong W. (1992). Writing is a technology that restructures thought. In: Dowling P. (ed.) *The Linguistics of Literacy*. Amsterdam: Benjamins, 293–319.

Zinck-Pedersen K. (2018) *Organising Patient Safety: Failsafe Fantasies and Pragmatic Practices*. London: Palgrave Macmillan.

Pink S. (2007) *Doing Visual Ethnography: Images, Media and Representation in Research*. London: Sage.

Prasad V, Vandross A, Toomey C, et al. (2013) A decade of reversal: An analysis of 146 contradicted medical practices. *Mayo Clinic Proceedings* 357: 790–798.

Prigogine I. (1996) *The End of Certainty: Time, Chaos and the New Laws of Nature.* New York: The Free Press.

Prigogine I and Stengers I. (1984) *Order Out of Chaos: Man's New Dialogue with Nature.* New York: Bantam.

Shekelle PG, Wachter RM, Pronovost PJ, et al. (2013) *Making Health Care Safer II: An Updated Critical Analysis of the Evidence for Patient Safety Practices.* Comparative Effectiveness Review No. 211. (Prepared by the Southern California-RAND Evidence-based Practice Center under Contract No. 290–2007–10062-I.) (AHRQ Publication No. 13-E001-EF.), Rockville, MD: Agency for Healthcare Research and Quality.

Shusterman R. (2008) *Body Consciousness: A Philosophy of Mindfulness and Somaesthetics.* Cambridge: Cambridge University Press.

Sloterdijk P. (1983) *Critique of Cynical Reason.* Minneapolis: University of Minnesota Press.

Sloterdijk P. (2009) *Du mußt dein Leben ändern: Über Anthropotechnik.* Frankfurt am Main: Suhrkamp.

West M and Lyubovnikova J. (2012) Real teams or pseudo teams? The changing landscape needs a better map. *Industrial and Organizational Psychology* 5: 25–55.

Wilden A. (1980) *System and Structure: Essays in Communication and Exchange.* London: Tavistock.

Wilden A. (1987) *The Rules Are No Game: The Strategy of Communication.* London: Routledge & Kegan Paul.

Wittgenstein L. (1953) *Philosophical Investigations.* Oxford: Blackwell.

Woods DD. (2006) Essential characteristics of resilience. In: Hollnagel E, Woods DD and Leveson N (eds) *Resilience Engineering: Concepts and Precepts.* Aldershot: Ashgate, 21–34.

Yu A, Flott K, Chainani N, et al. (2016) *Patient Safety 2030.* London: NIHR Imperial Patient Safety Translational Research Centre.

Appendix A: Examples of funded VRE projects

This appendix includes two examples of VRE project proposals that have attracted research funding. The first proposal was awarded funding to strengthen handover communication between ambulance and emergency department staff. The second proposal was awarded funding to investigate the more theoretical question about whether and how healthcare professional staff were managing the rising complexity of clinical care provision.

PROJECT TITLE: IMPROVING CLINICAL HANDOVER BETWEEN AMBULANCE OFFICERS AND EMERGENCY DEPARTMENT CLINICIANS USING 'FLEXIBLE STANDARDIZATION'

Summary of the proposed research

Aim: This project seeks to align handover processes between ambulance and emergency department (ED) staff with the NSW Health Safe Clinical Handover key principles.[1]

Objectives:
1. To engage ambulance and ED clinicians in assessment of and reflection on *real-time* visual data.
2. To design an *ambulance–ED handover standard/protocol* that aligns with the NSW Health Safe Clinical Handover key principles.[1]
3. To *integrate* this ambulance–ED handover standard/protocol *into practice*.
4. To *evaluate* how clinicians' use of the designed standard/protocol *adheres* to the NSW Health Safe Clinical Handover key principles.
5. To *evaluate the practical impact* of the designed standard/protocol on clinical safety.
6. To produce *e-learning tools* from this work to assist ambulance and ED staff across NSW.

Project background

An effective handover between ambulance staff and ED personnel is critical to ensuring all information critical to the patient's care is appropriately transferred.[2] Handover works when the expectations of ambulance staff and ED clinicians are aligned.[3] Aligning these expectations occurs through standardizing handover as outlined in the NSW Health Safe Clinical Handover key principles.[1] With a standardized handover, ambulance staff can prepare for what to hand over, and clinicians will be familiar with the general outline of what they will hear, and know what to ask for in addition in specific circumstances.

Focusing on ambulance-to-ED handover, this project extends work recently completed for the *Australian Commission on Safety and Quality in Health Care*. This work was part of the *Australian Commission on Safety and Quality in Health Care National Clinical Handover Project*. This work resulted in a range of international publications,[4,5] training resources,[6,7] handover improvement collaborations (e.g. with seven hospitals in the Netherlands) and workshop and lecture invitations.[1]

Methods

This study combines research with a handover practice intervention. The study deploys a before-and-after study design. Existing practice will be captured using interviews, focus groups as well as video. This practice will then be scrutinized by involving the staff themselves in its analysis. This reflexive process generates learning: our research has shown this process gives front-line staff an insight into why current practice is inadequate and into how practice should be redesigned.[4,5]

This learning process will be guided by the NSW Health Safe Clinical Handover key principles and will enable ambulance and ED staff to develop an NSW Health policy-compatible handover standard. The study method consists of the following:

1. *Participation*: Ambulance and ED staff will be involved through interviews and focus groups in outlining their concerns about existing handover practice and help define the *principal touch points*.[2]
2. *Observation*: Existing handover practice will be observed by a researcher to locate the principal touch points in real-time practice in preparation for filming.
3. *Filming*: Real-time handover will be captured on film as a way of making the principal touch points visible.

---

[1] Workshops: *BMJ – IHI International Forum on Quality and Safety in Health Care* (Paris 2008); *ACSQHC National Clinical Handover Symposia* 2008/9. Talks: Utrecht University Medical Centre & Dutch Patient Safety Centre (19 Feb & 26 Nov 2009); UK Health Foundation (12-16 April 2010) and University of Michigan (9 April 2010).

[2] A 'touchpoint' is a facet of practice that study participants and researchers identify as problematic and in need of attention and redesign.[8]

4. *Reflexive sessions*: Ambulance and ED staff will be involved in mixed focus groups to confront real-time practice, generate learning and derive insight into how to redesign handover into an NSW Health policy-compatible handover standard.
5. *Implementation*: Ambulance and ED staff will be involved in, first, simulated trials of the new handover standard and, second, real-time roll-out.
6. *Ongoing self-evaluation*: Ambulance and ED staff will be engaged in ongoing self-evaluation.[3]
7. *Dissemination and training*: Dissemination of the process leading to the production of the handover standard and the handover standard itself will occur by deploying video resources for general training and by involving front-line staff in training sessions at other hospital sites.

Evaluating the new handover standard

This study deploys a *before-and-after handover comparative evaluation*. This evaluation deploys the following criteria:

- *Degree of handover standardization* achieved by this intervention study
- *Relative frequency of patient management adjustments* brought about by the new standardized handover practice
- *Relative frequency of minor and major incidents* associated with the new standardized handover practice
- *Level of clinician confidence in their knowledge* about patients following the introduction of the new standardized handover practice
- *Level of patient satisfaction with information handling* (information involving them and information processes between clinicians and teams) as a result of the new standardized handover practice

The comparative evaluation methods include the following:

- *Document comparative evaluation*[4]: ambulance case sheet versus medical record comparison and analysis (targeting the transfer of information about, e.g. allergies, anti-coagulants and ambulance protocol [glyceryl trinitrate, chest pain])
- *Ethnographic comparative evaluation*: observational (ethnographic) analysis and filmed handover practice

---

[3] For example, through engaging junior staff in observational measurements for their clinical assessments, educationally supervised by their university.

[4] The document and ethnographic comparative evaluation will collectively gauge handover effectiveness and handover improvement post-standardization focusing on, among others, vital signs, medication information, severe sepsis and septic shock, confirmation of endotracheal tube placement, anticoagulation for acute pulmonary embolus patients, median time to fibrinolysis and median time to electrocardiogram.

- *Survey-based comparative evaluation*: questionnaire survey targeting the receiving team about their needs and views of the (changed) handover process

The dimensions of the study that will be evaluated include the following:

- The handover (re)design process ('was there learning?')
- The handover standard ('is it consistent with NSW Health policy?')
- The implementation of the handover standard ('does it produce better handover and safer care?')

Deliverables

The *deliverables* of this study are as follows:

- *Standardized handover practice* between ambulance and ED staff at the two participating sites: Prince of Wales and Royal Prince Alfred Hospitals
- *Comprehensive evaluation* of the standardized handover practice including the following:
  - Identification of adherence to the NSW Health Safe Clinical Handover key principles
  - Practical impact and success factors
- *A handover improvement resource* that brings together knowledge needed to standardize handover, including visual (video) records of standardized practice for induction and training purposes
- *International publications* into the academic literature co-authored by research investigators, policy makers and health department staff and local site clinical champions.

Theoretical background of the project

The literature shows there are now numerous clinical handover solutions, including SBAR, SIGNOUT, I PASS THE BATON and FIVE-Ps, among numerous others. Solutions such as these are proliferating without significantly or comprehensively impacting on front-line practice.[9]

Handover protocols and checklists find limited traction with front-line clinicians and teams.[9] This may be because staff are not assisted with deploying new handover solutions. Specifically, staff are not shown how to connect everyday practice to formally structured handover solutions.[4]

The approach available for connecting *in situ* practice to formal standards is termed 'flexible standardization'.[1] Flexible standardization involves front-line staff in confronting existing practice and in designing 'bottom-up' practice standards through participating in this reflexive process.[10] Thus, flexible standardization refers to the processes of involving clinicians in designing standards for communication by reflecting on real-time practice and in deploying and iteratively evaluating these standards.

In essence, flexible standardization requires clinicians to take time out from everyday (handover) practice, take stock of existing (handover) practice by producing data about it and develop ways of restructuring the (handover) practice and evaluating the improvements thus produced.

However, staff often lack the means, the people and the time to reflect on existing handover practice. Moreover, they often lack a language for negotiating handover options and adaptations. Further, their particular specialty or service may harbour unique constraints with regard to staff skill mix, patient portfolio complexity and information–knowledge sharing and storage technologies.

These factors indicate that what is called for is a study intervention that facilitates the process of front-line staff standardizing their handover practice. The handover practice improvement resource *HELiCS: Handover – Enabling Learning in Communication for Safety*[4] provides such a study intervention and will be deployed in the present intervention study.

Potential issues and constraints

It will be critical for this study to collaborate and align with existing NSW Health Clinical Handover projects. It will be equally necessary for this study to distinguish itself from these projects. This study is not just descriptive and analytical using social scientific disciplinary insights. Instead, this study is interventionist and focused on producing improved clinical outcomes. It involves front-line staff in learning about handover, standardizing handover, improving their communication practice and disseminating their learning through video resources, peer support and mentoring and other educational opportunities.

REFERENCES

1. NSW Health (2009) *The NSW Health Clinical Handover Toolkit*. Sydney, NSW: NSW Department of Health.
2. Thakore S, Morrison W (2001) A survey of the perceived quality of patient handover by ambulance staff in the resuscitation room. *Emer Med J* 18(2001):293–296.
3. London Ambulance Service (2008) *Procedure Relating to the Clinical Handover of Patients*. London: National Health Service UK.
4. Iedema R, Merrick E, Kerridge R, Herkes R, Lee B, Anscombe M, et al. (2009) 'Handover – Enabling Learning in Communication for Safety' (HELiCS): A report on achievements at two hospital sites. *Med J Aust* 190(11):S133–S136.
5. Iedema R, Merrick E, Rajbhandari D, Gardo A, Stirling A, Herkes R (2009) Viewing the taken-for-granted from under a different aspect: A video-based method in pursuit of patient safety. *Int J Mult Res Approaches* 3(3):290–301.
6. Iedema R, Merrick E (2008) *'Handover – Enabling Learning in Communication for Safety' (HELiCS)' – A DVD/Booklet-based Kit for*

Handover Improvement. Sydney, NSW: Australian Commission on Safety and Quality in Health Care & University of Technology Sydney.

7. Iedema R, Merrick E, Daly B, Thomas V (2009) Telling it like it is: People's experiences of an Emergency Department (DVD, 20 mins). Australia, University of Technology Sydney: Centre for Health Communication.

8. Bate P, Robert G (2007) *Bringing User Experience to Healthcare Improvement: The Concepts, Methods and Practices of Experience-Based Design*. Oxford/ Seattle, WA: Radcliffe Publishing.

9. Cohen M, Hilligoss B (2009) *Handoffs in Hospitals: A Review of the Literature on Information Exchange While Transferring Patient Responsibility or Control*. Ann Arbor: University of Michigan.

10. Timmermans S, Berg M (2003) *The Gold Standard: The Challenge of Evidence-Based Medicine and Standardization in Health Care*. Philadelphia, PA: Temple University Press.

PROJECT TITLE: PREVENTIVE HEALTHCARE: IS THE IDENTITY AND PRACTICE OF CLINICIANS ALIGNED WITH THE DIRECTION OF HEALTHCARE REFORM AND THE NEW ROLES IMPLIED IN ITS ACHIEVEMENT?

Aims and background

AIMS

This project has three overarching aims. First, the study seeks to examine and assess the extent to which healthcare workers are prepared for the intensification of organizational participation inherent in the reforms with which they are being confronted by policy makers, health organization managers and patients. Second, the study seeks to explore ways for staff to reflect on the substance of their work through their review of video data about their work. Third, the study seeks to refine videotaping as a method of organizational and work practice research.

BACKGROUND

The importance of a study which examines the way healthcare workers are affected by, respond to and are changing in respect of health reform initiatives cannot be underestimated. Policy makers and managements often take it for granted that there will be change on the ground in terms of workplace conducts, but the evidence about whether and how this is taking place is patchy.[1] The work of healthcare workers, as a subset of a larger workforce demographic we call 'professionals', does appear to be changing in 'post-bureaucratic' ways.[2,3] These people are required to be more involved in operational and strategic decision-making, be incorporated into workplace processes which no longer set clear distinctions between managerial prerogatives and worker obligations and show evidence of their 'empowerment'.[4] Generally seen as prominent in this context are participatory structures[5] and bottom-up solutions to problems.[6]

In general, however, research that enquires into employees' and managements' acceptance and implementation of work restructuring has rarely strayed beyond instrumental-mechanistic, cognistivist, critical-political or legal-ethical definitions of change. This study takes 'situated interaction' as its unit of analysis, and therefore transcends aforementioned approaches in three ways. First, this study focuses on *in situ* practice and on practitioners' reviews of these practices, and not on decontextualized and abstract descriptions, or considered and espoused views. Second, this study locates itself at the interstice between reform, identity and *in situ* practice, by filming what practitioners do and by getting them to review the resulting data. Third, the study is realized using an innovative methodological tool: video review analysis.

The rationale underpinning the study is that individual organizational reform initiatives in health increasingly ask employees to intensify,[7] objectify[8] and redesign[9] work. Earlier reform initiatives were about bureaucratization (rule- and regulation-oriented change) and managerialization (finance- and budget-oriented change) – initiatives which left employees to a greater or lesser extent untouched. By contrast, more recent reforms are 'simultaneously ... individualizing and totalizing',[10] that is, weaving individuals into organization-wide, policy-oriented conducts whose emergent organizational logic is comprised of *knowledging*,[11,12] *boundary spanning*,[13] and *participating*.[2,14] This emergent logic has been referred to as 'textualization'.[8,15] Textualization encompasses employees more and more frequently being called on to negotiate and act according to objectifying and codifying descriptions about their work, for the purposes of standardizing, benchmarking and coordinating services across specializations, disciplines and organizations. The success of this new ethos of work currently being foisted on staff depends on employees' ability and willingness to participate more intensely across a range of organizational fora where they, besides doing their work in more highly self-conscious ways, are to conduct discourses that acknowledge the right of multiple stakeholders to know about and have a say in their work.[16]

A second rationale underpinning the focus and design of this study is that textualization implicates people's professional self. Textualizing about work means employees (have to) distance themselves from those discourses, practices and positionings that have thus far anchored their professional 'identity'.[17] No longer 'a given, but a task',[18] employees' identity is less and less a stable and lasting effect of training and certification, and is becoming increasingly contingent upon the enactment[19] of the abovementioned stakeholder tensions and dynamics. Being 'response-ible', here, means devising and upholding locally achieved understandings, as well as framing these understandings in boundary spanning and objectifying discourses.[21] Put differently, 'response-ible' people engage in constant shunting between the local (teams, meetings) and the distal (data produced about the work, pathways and other formalized standardizations). Having to enact this responsibility (read: 'responsiveness') both at the 'clinical coal face' and in formal meeting rooms, employees are faced with putting their sense of practice and of truth, and thus both their public and private self, *at risk*.[9] As this 'responsibility' imposes 'new ways of being and doing at work',[20] it is central that we study how people negotiate work and change with one another *in situ*.

Hence, our research strategy centres on the implications for worker 'self' of this intensification in work participation, that is, on the professional and personal risks such participative and 'responsive' conduct incurs for employees and potentially patients. Focusing on the degree to which people assume such responsive conducts, the study adopts the notion 'textualization' as analytical lens for appraising organizational practices centred around cross-boundary participation and knowledging. Textualization enables this study to enquire into processes and interactions through which people 'distalize the local and localize the distal', or shift back and forth between 'what they do' and 'how work can be represented to others'.

This textualizing, as knowledging or 'discourse work', will bring to the fore the ethical, accountability and organizational contradictions inherent in traditional notions of professional identity as embodied in clinical autonomy, and reform as embodied in organizational participation and performance accountability. If clinicians are to move from a profession-centred to an organization-centred orientation, a shift in professional identity must take place. For instance, ethical dilemmas arise as clinician decision-making moves from the interests of individual patients to patient populations, where immediate clinical decisions impact on resource availability and the capacity to service future and, as yet, unknown patient needs. Accountability dilemmas occur as traditional notions of opaque individual clinician accountability for performance transform into scrutiny by multiple stakeholders of transparent and open reporting systems. Dilemmas about organization emerge as clinicians make the transition from individual practitioner diagnostic and therapeutic preferences to collective, multidisciplinary, systematized and standardized ways of managing clinical work. In each of these situations, local experiences are, or are not, textualized into distal representations, languages, concerns and codes.

It is in this way that the detail of reform requires a far-reaching re-fashioning of clinical identity and conduct from that of a self-responsible individual practitioner to a collective-responsible organizational player. This transition in identity and conduct will encourage clinicians, particularly medical clinicians, to regroup in a way that may detach loyalty from a specialty/subspecialty and to re-form as part of a local 'team'. This regrouping will alter traditional affiliations based principally on disciplines, – i.e. 'doctors and nurses', 'clinicians and managers', to a more locally-based affiliation, such as 'team', 'product' or 'service'. Such transition in affiliation impacts on clinician identity and positioning in two ways. First, the development of representational processes among clinicians, medical clinicians in particular, about clinical work management will encourage a *coalescence* of clinico-organizational interests. Second, and relatedly, clinicians may find more in common with managers within an emerging organizational logic as joint interests emerge around local issues. Inevitably, cleavage lines will re-form along local versus regional interests, diminishing functional and disciplinary divisions.

In the light of this, we ask, What is the process involved in identity and conduct change? How does this process manifest in the interactive (re)positioning of clinicians? What does it mean for them to undertake new roles, and how does 'identity-in-transition' impact on relationships with patients, with peers, with profession, with colleagues and with organization? At a more technical level, about the way they speak, self-present and act, we ask, What kinds of boundary settings and/or boundary spannings do they speak and act into being? Do they speak for and with people other than the original peer group? Do they produce boundary-spanning *talk* in conjunction with other boundary-spanning conducts? Finally, do they translate these conducts and ways of being into other media, as co-produced writing, data, designs or other meta-discursive schemas that then serve as shorthands for these new under-standings and agreements?

This study investigates these questions using video data. Videotaping has been used to great advantage in health and in other industries as a means for analysis of how employees communicate and interact. Unique to this study, the videotap-ing serves three objectives. First, it reveals to employees themselves their conduct and its logics, to enable them to revisit and re-fashion taken-as-given aspects and routines of work and self. In this way, the study seeks to induce in people the sense of being objectified and gets them to engage with 'textualizing' work and self. Such objectification may enhance reflexivity beyond what is achievable on the strength of interviews and other purely linguistically based kinds of enquiry. Second, the study investigates people's accounts produced during these video reviews as conduct displays seeking closure or allowing textualization. In this way, the study avoids relying on considered kinds of 'self-reports' only yielding decontextualized, espoused and habituated forms of talk as is typical of inter-views, focus groups and surveys. Third, the study analyses video data as records of embodied conduct *in situ*.

RELATIONSHIP TO THE FIELD

Preventive health care is health care that is structured so as to obviate the occur-rence of health problems in populations. One dimension of such preventive care is health promotion; another is the safe and risk-free organization of healthcare provision.[22] Safe and high-quality health care is dependent on workers being able to develop their new role and the identities that buttress their new role. This involves not merely clinicians accepting but *promoting* the development of performance monitoring and management systems, evaluation of outcomes, evidence-based clinical practice, clinical management roles and so on. In con-junction with clinicians moving from a curative to a preventive focus, then, pre-ventive care involves people's ability to move more flexibly between individual patients' pathology and a population-based wellness model.[23,24]

In Australia as well as overseas, the pursuit of preventive approaches to securing safe, high-quality and risk-free clinical work has produced a litany of organizational change initiatives. Among these, the most recent emphasizes performance contracting, purchaser–provider relationships, continuity of care, integrated services, coordinated care, clinical governance, clinical pathways, consumer involvement, clinical practice improvement, multidisciplinary teams, benchmarking, safety and quality initiatives and, last but not least, the digiti-zation of data gathering and networking of information processing, enhancing intra- and inter-organizational communication and monitoring. These reform initiatives have had a dramatic impact on the daily practices of ordinary employees, with the most frequently observed complaint touching on the ballooning of administrative and pseudo-managerial tasks in people's everyday working lives.[25,26]

Each of the organizational change initiatives detailed above impinges on clinicians' perception of self and practice. The interconnection between organizational change initiatives and performance of self is exemplified in performance contracting. Here, the pervasiveness of reform and its intrusion into clinical domains and everyday practice is directly influenced, for instance, by the market and principal–agent relationships embodied in notions of public choice designed to reduce risk and moral hazard. Here, preventive health care, and evidence of its attainment, cannot be separated from 'performance'.[27] While considering the relationship between improvement and performance, the relationship between identity and autonomy, legal obligation and professional ethics, and organization reform also needs to be considered. For example, the increasing formalization and explicitness of performance expectations for health services, for individual managers and for some practitioners, such as service agreements, individual performance agreements and visiting medical officer work contracts, bring into play the new role(s) envisaged for clinicians as embodied in legal contractual arrangements. Meeting financial and quality performance expectations entails increasing participation of clinicians in bureaucratic organizational processes that standardize, systematize and collectivize clinical work and clinical accountability in ways that are at odds with current professional conceptions of autonomy, independence, practice methods and identity. As these tensions are played out in interaction, people will either resist or become reflexive about their new roles and identities. Their reflexivity may result in unlearning and re-learning who they are and what they do, or what Argyris[28] has referred to as 'double-loop learning'. In engaging employees with their own objectification by means of video footage, this study empiricizes not only the enactment of reform processes but also the unlearning/re-learning upon which such reform is contingent.

Bringing together reform, identity and situated practice, this study operates on the outside of mainstream research agendas. By and large, the tools used for studying organizational change remain insensitive to the nexus of situated practice and the performative dimensions of employees' organizational relationships and identity. This is because most research into organizational reform glosses over these matters in favour of rational-instrumental,[29] cognitivist-psychoanalytical,[30] (sub)cultural,[31,32] legal-calculative[33] or narrative-based conceptions of change.[34] Such approaches all lack the means to study the situated performance of self and work relationships, reducing people and their interactive relationships to personality categories, cultural characteristics, open-ended narratives and out-of-context monologues or standardized and predetermined survey answers. While recent research has begun to pay more attention to social practice,[35] the analyses associated with this strand of research[36] predominantly focus on the micro-instrumental dimensions of practice[37,38] and have so far addressed only in a very limited way how situated practices answer to, or are bending under the weight of, organizational reform.

In contrast to those research approaches, then, this study homes in on the interstices between situated enactment, reform and identity: '[p]recisely because identities are constructed within, not outside, discourse, we need to understand them as produced in specific discursive formations and practices, by specific enunciative strategies',[39,40] such as performance contracting. In creating a context for practitioners where they can review and reconsider situated interaction, and where they can reflect on the interstice between identity, situated practice and reform, we can study how people discourse about their work and work relationships, and ask whether and how people manage to adopt and display the boundary-spanning ways of doing and being that are the crux of organizational reform. We believe we need such focus on situated conduct, because it is that which we as researchers *and* as employees need to question and rethink. Only a focus on situated conduct will enable us to assess and reconfigure the implications for and impact on work and workers of rising levels of participation, textualization and knowledging.

The thesis that drives this study, then, is that by getting employees to review and comment on their 'self-in-practice', they are better able to reconfigure their professional and emotional investments in particular ways of doing and being, and come to terms with having to display a 'flexibilized self'.[14] Aside from healthcare, aviation is a domain where employees' situated conducts have had the benefit of observation, questioning and re-fashioning.[41] With their primary concern being the safety and risk management strategies of cockpit personnel, aviation experts have introduced techniques that enable the review of professionals' conducts. Prominent among these, the videotaping of ordinary work tasks has played a crucial role in enabling practitioner professionals to observe *post hoc*, and through that reflect on their conducts in relation to others and their work. This study sees providing employees with such a meta-perspective on themselves as a crucial means for encouraging them to reflect on their work and work relationships. By gaining distance from the work in this way, employees may be able to re-frame work and self through experimenting with alternative ways of doing, being and saying, and in that way achieve personal, professional and organizational learning. By the same token, neither reform nor research here is 'done to', but 'done with'.

Significance and innovation

It is hard to overstate the significance of this study with regard to both its orientation towards organizational change research and the applicability of its findings to other situations. Its innovative nature resides in its design of methodology.

The significance of this study is, first, that it seeks to empiricize the proposition that employees (are to) negotiate their work procedures and relationships in increasingly 'self-organizing' ways. In addition, and due to the technization of work,[42] this also involves exchanging and translating details about their work into meta-discourses and abstract codes. This research is crucial because little attention has been paid to the interactive dimension of such emergent, 'post-bureaucratic' forms of work.

A second point of significance is that this study has two main prongs: it analyzes employees' interactions, and it investigates the potential and the unfolding of reflexivity by involving employees in the review and scrutiny of video data about those interactions. The former analysis will enhance our understanding of the impact on people's practices of the various reform imperatives, and of those conducts that realize the boundary-spanning, risk-taking and identity-reconfiguring conducts upon which organizational reform is contingent. With respect to the latter, the video review sessions are assessed in terms of their impact on people's technical, social, systemic and personal insight into what they do and who they are, measured on the strength of the discourse that they produce in response to the viewings. Isolated studies in trauma care have shown the power of using video data to engender reflection on specific care practices,[43,44] but only recently has video research been recognized as a powerful method for focusing on quality and safety.[41] A novel way to deepen and widen the research record, this study develops Helmreich's work, seeking not merely to engender reflexivity but to *understand its unfolding*.

Third, the study will highlight power relationships within the organization that may show, among other things, that people are so stressed that they either won't or can't respond to reform as envisaged in policy, or that they are attempting to change their practices but within an unresponsive management environment. This particular scenario will have major repercussions for policy development and implementation. It would seek to embolden the rhetoric of reform policy with an evidence base.

Finally, the project will produce insights that are of considerable value in health education, with a specific focus on the interpersonal and inter professional dimensions of practice. A fine-grained understanding of practitioners' interactions will provide insight not only into factors that support and undermine the introduction of new work practices and policies in clinical settings, but also into the emergence of bottom-up creative responses and their translation into workplace policies and organizational knowledge.

Approach

The three abovementioned aims each comprise a number of specific objectives. The first aim – to assess the extent to which healthcare workers are prepared for the impending intensification of organizational participation inherent in reform – is to be realized by the following four objectives. The study undertakes the following:

1. To produce an objective map of the work in terms of skill mixes, staff turnover, casemix, and various other administrative and organizational characteristics.
2. Following ethnographic exploration and enrolment of practitioners on site, to videotape employees doing their work.
3. To share with employees selected video data about their day-to-day work practices, and elicit accounts while people watch and review the video data. Accounts will be elicited about the work process or systems level and about the micro or situated level. These accounts will be transcribed.

4. To analyze whether and the ways in which people justify or rethink their (interactive) work practices during their accounts produced in response to watching the videos. Analysis will focus on people's interactive positionings, and the discursive-semiotic means they mobilize for realizing and maintaining, or questioning and potentially spanning boundaries.

The second aim – to enhance staff's preparedness for and commitment to reform – will be realized by means of the following three objectives. The study undertakes the following:

1. To encourage people to reflect on who they are and what they do through video review, and to guide them towards new understandings about self and practice both privately and in group situations. The protocol for this phase of the research will be elaborated from earlier work,[45,46] and it will be facilitated with close involvement of the chief investigators.
2. To explore with employees our analyses of their accounts about the video data.
3. To facilitate employees' production of formative and summative observations about the achievements and benefits of the study.

The third aim – to refine video research as a means to achieving organizational and work practice change – is realized by the following two objectives. The study undertakes the following:

1. To elaborate practice and analysis protocols for the video review phase of the research where most of the reflection and 'change work' is to be achieved.
2. To subject extant video analyses of workplace conduct to interrogation and emulate video-based research procedures and understandings.

FRAMEWORK AND DESIGN

To achieve the above aims, the study comprises an embedded multiple case study design.[47] First, there is a research strand that maps the 'objective' characteristics of the sites focusing on administrative and organizational characteristics such as casemix, skill mix, staff turnover, types of meetings and modes of record keeping. Embedded in this are video case studies and the 'objective' analysis of the video data, 'subjective' account production by employees on reviewing that data intertwined with elicitation and guidance, and again 'objective' analysis of these accounts. The videotaping will focus on the domains of work identified as 'hot spots' but negotiated with employees, e.g. ward rounds, negotiating decisions across professions, notating clinical decisions, effecting practice changes and negotiating decisions with patients and carers.

Three full-time researchers will conduct the video recording and feedback sessions at the sites: a research associate, an Australian Post-Graduate Award PhD student and a research assistant level 7 (RA). The PhD student is additionally responsible for the analysis of the video material using semiotics (see below). The chief investigators will be closely involved in structuring the research, organizing and facilitating the feedback meetings and disseminating results. The RA will focus on the formal mapping of the sites' characteristics and their analysis, and the PhD student and the research associate will be in charge of video recording, organizing the video replay sessions and analyzing the accounts produced during these replay sessions.

The study will unfold in *nine* phases during the course of the 3 years in accordance with the aims and objectives set out earlier. Some iteration and overlap is expected between these phases. *Phase 1* of the study *(Jan–Mar '04)* will assemble a reference group comprising the study's investigators and consultants (see below) together with researchers and clinicians with common interests. The reference will monitor the progress of the study, assess its achievements and provide guidance and advice as to decisions and directions taken. During this phase, ethics approval will be sought, and any necessary negotiations with the cooperating institutions will be completed. *Phase 2 (Apr–Jun '04)* initiates the research, with the RA profiling the relevant sites and the other two researchers starting their ethnographic explorations and arranging for the filming. Provisional consent for filming is secured at the level of the clinical investigators named in this grant and will need to be pursued with the personnel of their units, the ethics committees of their hospitals and the ethics committee at the University of New South Wales. *Phase 3 (Jul–Dec '04)* is comprised of the videoing of the clinical work. The purpose here is to obtain representative stretches of practice on film. *Phase 4 (Jan–Jun '05)* centres on the elicitation from practitioners of accounts about the video data and our guidance into their potential reflexivity about self and practice. During *Phase 5 (Jul–Oct '05)*, these accounts will be transcribed and analyzed, with the aim of illuminating their boundary-spanning versus boundary-maintaining characteristics. At this point, the PhD student will branch off from the main study and deploy social semiotic analysis to selected aspects of the video material. This PhD student will emulate analytical procedures of enquiry laid down in the domains of 'qualitative ethology'[46] and 'workplace studies'.[37,38,48-50] During *Phase 6 (Nov '05)*, there will be feedback of findings to practitioners to test, negotiate and re-frame our analytical and summative observations. Phase 4 provides occasion for practitioners to reflect on and/or justify their conducts, whereas Phase 6 provides occasion for the researchers to present, negotiate and reshape *their* observations and understandings. *Phase 7 (Dec '05–Jan '06)* synthesizes the study and outlines its overall results. *Phase 8 (Jan–Feb '06)* evaluates the study against the aims that it has set itself. *Phase 9 (Feb–Dec '06)* focuses on result dissemination (see E6). The table sets these phases out in terms of responsibilities, outputs and projected timeline.

Methods

WEEKLY MEETINGS AND MEMO EXCHANGE BETWEEN RESEARCHERS AND INVESTIGATORS

Collaboration between researchers and investigators will occur throughout the whole study by exchange of written research memos and open discussions at half-day weekly meetings, to critically appraise all aspects of the study as it develops. Since the investigators and researchers bring methods from different disciplines to bear in the analysis (medicine, nursing, management and organization theory, discourse and semiotic analysis), this process will constitute a form of triangulation.

FORMAL ORGANIZATIONAL PROFILING

The organizational profiling process will capture organizational and systems-wide available data including staffing profiles and skill mix, service profile, organizational structure, existing process indicators and current information and communication technologies. Documentation sought will be available from active databases, annual reports, structure charts, internal reports and other administrative data.

VIDEOTAPING

The videotaping will involve filming the relevant aspects of work practice as identified through non-participant observation and in negotiation with practitioners. In this study, video data will serve two purposes. First, they will serve as springboard for employees to produce accounts about their self in practice (see below). Second, explained further below, the video data will be analyzed by the investigators using micro-behavioural analytic methods. Thus, the video data serve both as cues for reflection and as analytical materials, enabling subjective and objective explorations of work and workers. Overall, this video component is innovative because it becomes the point of convergence for detailed attention given to work practices and interactive dynamics and an analysis of policy implementation.[51]

VIDEOTAPE REVIEW PROCESS

Video recordings often provide analytical material for researchers only.[52] It has been recognized, however, that reviewing videotapes of 'self in practice' can be beneficial.[43-46] Employees' account giving while reviewing video data offers them the opportunity for reflecting on and distancing themselves from accepted ways of doing and being. We are aware that asking clinicians to view, reflect and comment on their own conduct may be confronting, and that they will respond in myriad different ways. Here, self-image will come into play, as well as the impact of their intervention on the patient (were messages clearly understood), the effect of their communications with colleagues (did they get the level of cooperation required) and so on. For this reason, this dimension of the study is likely to operate at a number of levels that assess the ability of participants to evaluate and to objectify their own conduct as a method of learning and practice change. Closely involved with this part of the study, CI2 and CI3 have extensive experience and qualifications in change management facilitation and counseling.

ACCOUNT ANALYSIS

Approximately 40 accounts (20 in the primary site and 10 in each secondary site) each of 30–60 min duration will be elicited. This number permits pinpointing of discursive variation both within and between the different groups of practitioners. These accounts will be analyzed not only for their substantive content ('what is talked about?') but also as *performances of self*.[19,53] This involves establishing to what extent the talk comes to question and reflect on, or uphold and legitimate particular ways of doing and being. The analysis will draw on two bodies of research work. First, it will draw on work done by the principal investigator (PI) into people's discursive performance. This work has illuminated the performative dimension of work[54] and the discursive nature of organizational information and communication strategies. The research will also draw on research that analyses accounts as *displays* of professional identity.[55]

VIDEO ANALYSIS (PHD)

Video analysis is comprised of the close transcription of behavioural sequences and outlines regularities at the level of social distance between interactants (proxemics), their bodily movements (kinesics), facial expressions and gestural signings, with a specific focus on higher order regularities in conduct and their relationship to organizational and policy issues. Producing an 'ethogram' using the work of Birdwhistell,[56] Kendon[57] and the more recent applications presented in Martinec,[58] this PhD will emulate the work currently characterizing fields such as 'qualitative ethology'[46] and 'workplace studies',[36] by integrating analyses of identity performance and organizational reform.

SITES

The work units we have chosen to involve in this study are teams working in high-pressure healthcare settings. Intensive care units and spinal injury units are particularly suited to this role as they present a context in which issues of commitment and participation are brought into sharp relief by extreme daily challenges to health, self and relationships.

FEASIBILITY AND SUPPORT FOR THE STUDY

This study is supported by medical, ethical and social scientific expertise, and feasible in terms of access to required sites and access to staff and participation within appropriate clinical units. The research centre is the Centre for Clinical Governance Research at the University of New South Wales. The primary site of the study will be John Hunter Hospital. This has been negotiated with clinical directors who will be the study's internal supervisors at that site. The researchers have also secured in-principle agreements from a secondary site. The involvement of two sites will strengthen the findings, as commonalities are identified and as differences are delineated and explained.

Methodologies similar to those proposed in this study are being employed in a study of digitization of clinical practice, involving the chief investigators. Synthesis between these efforts will not only facilitate a ready consultation process in supporting the development of methodology and understanding of the findings from this study but also create a capacity building momentum around groundbreaking research and organizational change methods.

ETHICAL CONSIDERATIONS

Informed consent from practitioners will be obtained for the purpose of videotaping and open-ended account giving sessions. Informed consent will also be sought from the director and staff of units for the video work. All data will be in digital form and will be de-identified and stored on a non-networked, password-protected computer. Patients will be approached for consent to interview only when the director of the unit indicates that this is appropriate, and if and when they become implicated in the videotaping. Staff will be reassured that non-participation will not incur deleterious consequences. Anonymity of staff participating in the videotaping and account giving will be guaranteed as much as possible to protect professional and organizational relationships. No identificatory research data will be put into the public domain. Video data will be securely kept within the Centre in a locked cabinet for the required period and destroyed according to university regulations after that time. All informants will be assigned pseudonyms, and quotes taken from the accounts for the purposes of illustration or publication will be altered so that no individuals can be identified. The videotaping, permission to video and provisos and limitations which attach to it will be negotiated with the relevant clinical and administrative staff.

NATIONAL BENEFIT

Appropriate and effective communication and coordination of work is central to safe and high-quality health care. The national benefit of this work is that it explores the impact of workplace reform on work. This is crucial because the participative intensity of work is likely to exacerbate, and many workers have no option other than to build new ways of being and doing with which to confront and negotiate previously impervious boundaries. Given that, and in addition to the rapid pace of social, organizational and technological change, tensions among social, cultural and professional groups are not merely counterproductive but destructive.[1] The study will shed light on the quality of the environment in which reform is being enacted and will highlight the role and effectiveness of hospital management in facilitating change, and the extent to which health reform policy is supportive and inclusive of those charged with its implementation. Homing in on tensions between the enactment of work and organizational reform, this study has importance for health policy and service organization at local, state and national levels.

Expected economic and social returns to the broader Australian community – The broader Australian community will benefit from more efficient and effective modes of healthcare work. It has been calculated that '16.6% of hospital admissions were associated with iatrogenic patient injury'[59] and that '[f]ifty percent of these adverse events were judged to have a high preventability score'. Further, it has been estimated that that improved work systems, that is, clinicians participating in knowledging and boundary spanning about their work, 'could save between 15% and 25% of our total cost of operations'.[60] Given these injury and prevention rates, it is economically and socially imperative to roll out improvements booked in the conduct of trauma care[43,44] and other areas of healthcare work.[41] Other research results show that up to 41% of patients admitted to the ICU had suboptimal care attributed to ineffective team processes.[61] Improving communication between clinicians, clinicians and management, and between clinical and organizational systems is likely to benefit patients and co-service providers. This study represents a first phase in assessing the readiness of organizations to enact reform in its focus on clinicians. Similar studies would be applicable to gauge the alignment of manager identity and practice with reform objectives.

Communication of results

Research findings will be tested as they emerge by presenting them to, and soliciting feedback from, the different stakeholder groups who are included in this study. Members of staff at the participating sites will be recruited as active contributors to the process of interpreting the data and revising the research findings. Those outside the clinical context (including the reference group) will be invited to consider the applicability of these findings to their settings and problematics.

REFERENCES

1. Sorensen R (2002) The Dilemma of Reform: Recognising the limits of policymaking, managerialism and professionalism as factors in reform. Unpublished PhD thesis. Sydney, NSW: UNSW.
2. Heckscher C (1994) Defining the post-bureaucratic type. Heckscher C, Donnellon A (eds.) *The Post-Bureaucratic Organization* (pp. 14–62). Thousand Oaks, CA: Sage.
3. Covaleski MA, Dirsmith MW, Heian JB, Samuel S (1998) The calculated and the avowed: Techniques of discipline and struggles over identity in big six public accounting firms. *ASQ* 43(2):293–327.
4. Lloyd P, Braithwaite J, Southon G (1999) Empowerment and the performance of health services. *J Man Med* 13(2):83–94.
5. Braithwaite J (1999) Incorporating medical clinicians into management: An examination of clinical directorates. Unpublished PhD thesis. Sydney, NSW: UNSW.
6. Senge PM (1990) *The Fifth Discipline*. Sydney, NSW: Random House.
7. Lyotard JF (1984) *The Postmodern Condition*. Minneapolis: University of Minnesota Press.
8. Darville R (1995) Literacy experience, knowledge and power. Campbell M, Manicom A (eds.) *Knowledge, Experience and Ruling Relations* (pp. 249–261). Toronto: University of Toronto Press.
9. Gee J (2000) Communities of practice in the new capitalism. *J Lear Sci.* 9(4):515–523.
10. Gordon C (1991) Introduction. Burchell G, Gordon C, Miller P (eds.) *The Foucault Effect: Studies in Governmentality* (pp. 1–51). Hemel Hampstead: Harvester Wheatsheaf.

11. Adler PS (2001) Market, hierarchy, and trust: The knowledge economy and the future of capitalism. *Org Sci.* 12(2) 215–234.
12. Child J, McGrath RG (2001) Organizations unfettered: Organizational form in an information-intensive economy. *Acad Man J* 44(6):1135–1148.
13. Ancona DG (1990) Outward bound: Strategies for team survival in the organization. *Acad Man J* 33:334–365.
14. Grey C, Garsten C (2001) Trust, control and post-bureaucracy. *Org Stud* 22(20):229–250.
15. Jackson N (2001) Writing up people at work: Investigations of workplace literacy. *Lit Num Stud* 10(1):1–18.
16. Gee JP, Hull G, Lankshear, C (1996) *The New Work Order.* Sydney, NSW: Allen & Unwin.
17. Harré R (1991) The discursive construction of the self. *Theor Psychol* 1(1):51–63.
18. Bauman Z (2001) *The Individualized Society.* Cambridge: Polity Press.
19. Butler J (1997) *Excitable Speech: A Politics of the Performative.* London: Routledge.
20. du Gay P (1996) *Consumption and Identity at Work.* London: Sage.
21. Iedema R (2003) The medical record as organising discourse. *Doc Des* 4(1):64–84.
22. Berwick D (1998) Developing and testing changes in delivery of care. *Ann Int Med* 128(8):651–656.
23. Davies C, Salvage J, Smith R (1999) Doctors and nurses: Changing family values. *BMJ* 319:463–464.
24. Doyal L, Cameron A (2000) Reshaping the NHS workforce. *BMJ* 320:1023–1024.
25. Latham L, Freeman T, Walshe K, Spurgeon P, Wallace L (2000) Clinical Governance in the West Midlands and South Wets regions: Early progress in NHS trusts. *Clin Man* 9:83–91.
26. Packwood T, Keen J, Buxton, M (1992) Process and structure: Resource management and the development of sub-unit organizational structure. *Health Serv Man Res* 5(1):66–76.
27. Creighton F, Bernard A, McMahon L (1990) An integrated inpatient management model. *Health Care Man* 15(1):61–70.
28. Argyris C (1994) Good communication that blocks learning. *Har Bus Rev* 72:77–85.
29. Edmondson A, Bohmer R, Pisano G (2001) Disrupted routines: Team learning and new technology implementation in hospitals. *ASQ* 46(2001):685–716.
30. Reciniello, S (1999) The emergence of a powerful female workforce as a threat to organizational identity: What psychoanalysis can offer. *Am Behav Sci* 43(2):301–323.
31. Hofstede GMN et al. (1990) Measuring organizational cultures: A qualitative and quantitative study across 20 cases. *ASQ* 35(2):286.
32. Degeling P, Kennedy J, Hill M (1998) Professional subcultures and hospital reform. *Clin Man* 7(2):89–98.

33. Blandford J, Smythe T (2002) From risk management to clinical governance. Harris M (ed.). *Managing Health Services* (pp. 378–401). Sydney, NSW: MacLennan and Petty.
34. Boje DM (2001) *Narrative Methods for Organizational & Communication Research*. London: Sage.
35. Wenger E (1998) *Communities of Practice*. Cambridge: CUP.
36. Engeström Y, Middleton D (1998) *Cognition and Communication at Work*. Cambridge: CUP.
37. Heath C, Luff P (1992) Media space and communicative asymmetries: Preliminary observations of video-mediated interaction. *Hum Comput Inter* 7(3):315–346.
38. Heath C, Luff P (1998) Convergent activities. Engeström Y, Middleton D (eds.) *Cognition and Communication at Work* (pp. 96–129). Cambridge: CUP.
39. Hall S (1996) Who needs identity? Hall S, du Gay P (eds.) *Questions of Cultural Identity* (pp. 1–17). London: Sage.
40. Rose N (1996) Identity, genealogy, history. Hall S, du Gay P (eds.) Questions of Cultural Identity (pp. 128–150). London: Sage.
41. Helmreich R (2000) On error management: Lessons from aviation. *BMJ* 320:781–785.
42. Barley S (1996) Technicians in the workplace: Ethnographic evidence for bringing work into organization studies. *ASQ* 41:404–441.
43. Santora T, Trooskin S, Blank C, Clarke J, Schinco M (1995) Video assessment of trauma response: Adherence to ATLS protocols. *Am J Emer Med* 14:564–569.
44. Michaelson M, Levi L (1997) Videotaping in the admitting area: A most useful tool for quality improvement of the trauma care. *Eur J Emerg Med* 4:94–96.
45. Engeström Y (1993) Developmental studies in work as a testbench of activity theory. Chaiklin S, Lave J (eds.) *Understanding Practice* (pp. 64–103). Cambridge: CUP.
46. Bottorff JL (1994) Using video-taped recordings in qualitative research. Morse J (ed.). *Critical Issues in Qualitative Research Methods* (pp. 244–61). Thousand Oaks, CA: Sage.
47. Eisenhardt K (1989) Building theories from case study research. *Acad Man Rev* 14:532–550.
48. Goodwin C, Goodwin M (1998) Seeing as situated activity. Engeström Y, Middleton D (eds.) *Cognition and Communication at Work* (pp. 61–95). Cambridge: CUP.
49. Hutchins E, Klausen T (1998) Distributed cognition in an airline cockpit. Engeström Y, Middleton D (eds.) *Cognition and Communication at Work* (pp. 15–34). Cambridge: CUP.
50. Engeström Y (1999) Expansive visibilization of work. *J Collab Comp* 8(1):63–93.
51. Strauss A (1987) *Qualitative Analysis for Social Scientists*. Cambridge: CUP.

52. Latvala E, Vuokila-Oikkonen P, Janhonen, S (2000) Video-taped recording as a method of participant observation in psychiatric nursing research. *J Adv Nurs* 31(5):1252–1257.

53. Butler J (1996) Performativity's social magic. Schatzki T, Natter W (eds.) *The Social and Political Body* (pp. 29–48). New York: The Guilford Press.

54. Iedema R, Degeling P (2001) Quality of care: Clinical governance and pathways. *AHR* 24(3):12–15.

55. Jordens C, Little M, Paul K, Sayers E (2001) Life disruption and generic complexity: a social linguistic analysis of narratives of cancer illness. *Soc Sci Med* 53(9):1227–1236.

56. Birdwhistell R (1970) *Kinesics and Context*. Harmondsworth: Penguin.

57. Kendon A (1990) *Conducting Interaction*. Cambridge: CUP.

58. Martinec R (2001) Interpersonal resources in action. *Semiotica* 135(1/4):117–145.

59. Wilson R, Harrison B, Gibberd R, Hamilton J (1999) An analysis of the causes of adverse events from the Quality in Australian Health Care Study. *MJA* 170:411–415.

60. James B (2002) *Minimising Harm to Patients in Hospital*. Sydney, NSW: Australian Broadcasting Corporation.

61. McQuillan P, Pilkington S (1998) Confidence inquiry into quality of care before admission to intensive care. *BMJ* 316:1853–1858.

Appendix B: VRE and ethics

This appendix elaborates on the ethical frameworks underpinning video-reflexive ethnography (VRE).

A SITUATED ETHICS APPROACH

A situated ethics approach (Clark, 2012; Clark, 2013; Gubrium et al,. 2013) recognizes that ethical decisions are context dependent rather than once and for all, or 'one size fits all'. Such approach considers visual ethical issues as part of an ongoing process of reflection and negotiation. 'A situational ethics approach recognizes that decisions are evaluated and made in the context of time and place as well as who is involved rather than according to a set of prescriptive rigid rules or regulations to be adhered to or wholly adopted' (Clark 2012, p. 25). This approach to decision-making is valid whether decisions are concerned with deciding what to film and what not to film, what to show back or not to show back and in what circumstances. Clark is keen to point out, however, that a situated visual ethics approach does not simply mean going with what a particular participant requests. Rather, it entails the researcher making decisions in collaboration with participants and giving due consideration to the context in which clips might be shown and how they might be seen and interpreted.

Wyer (2017) researched with patients and clinicians to explore the practical and relational complexities of patient involvement in infection prevention and control. Hospital inpatients viewed footage of their own clinical care to look for infection risks. The original footage of the care interaction was then shown to the nurses who cared for these patients, alongside patients' observations of the same footage. Some of the patients requested that footage be shown in which they were quite critical of particular clinicians (e.g. doctors or nurses) and/or aspects of care. This posed a dilemma for Wyer:

> I felt strongly that patients should drive what the nurses viewed in reflexive sessions. At the same time, as a nurse, and being involved in the larger project, I could also relate to the pressures these nurses were working under. A research aim was to enable relationships, so I did not wish to repeatedly confront staff with negative comments about their work in a way that might hinder their ability

to see and hear what patients had to say. Furthermore, I worried that the video messages some patients asked me to relay might have damaging effects for patient/provider relationships and/or care, particularly when the patient was still an inpatient or was likely to return for care in the future.

(Collier and Wyer 2016, p. 9)

Wyer responded to these situations by discussing her concerns with patients and sometimes planned, with them, a less confronting option for relaying messages to clinicians. When patients insisted that these more critical messages be delivered in a video format, Wyer ensured that during reflexive sessions, these kinds of clips were balanced with more positive or neutral accounts (Collier and Wyer 2016).

INDIGENOUS ETHICS FRAMEWORK

While none of us can claim to write from an indigenous position, we nevertheless recognize that the academy of which we are a part is defined by views of science and scholarship that privilege nonindigenous types of knowledge and ethics frameworks. Countervailing this, there is now a growing and significant body of literature questioning these methodologies and ethics frameworks. This alternative literature draws on indigenous approaches to research and research collaboration. Thus, Chatterji (2001) describes indigenous research as 'liberatory practice within postcolonial context that seeks to create knowledge relevant to the communities it purports to serve' (Chatterji 2001, p. 1). While by no means unified and entirely monological, indigenous ethics tends to agree that research be carried out in a participatory, respectful, ethical and beneficial manner (Gott et al. 2011).

In this 'nothing-about-us-without-us' paradigm, the researcher and participants are construed as setting out together in a particular direction, and perhaps sharing some general understandings about what is to occur, but as principally having to check in with one another constantly about how to structure the day-to-day research as such. As explained in our earlier work (Iedema et al. 2013), VRE aligns itself with the statements by indigenous scholars for guidance on how to approach matters of ethics, participation, outcomes and knowledge production. Specifically, indigenous research ethics are underpinned by collaboration, partnership and reciprocation. This overarching philosophical approach is set out in the introductory paragraphs of the Australian Guidelines for Ethical Research in Australian Indigenous Studies:

It is essential that Indigenous people are full participants in research projects that concern them, share an understanding of the aims and methods of the research, and share the results of this work. At every stage, research with and about Indigenous Peoples must be founded on a process of meaningful engagement and reciprocity between the researcher and Indigenous people. It should also be recognised that there is no sharp distinction between researchers and Indigenous people. Indigenous people are also researchers, and all participants must be regarded as equal participants in a research engagement.

(Australian Institute of Aboriginal and Torres Strait Islander Studies 2012)

Kaupapa Māori methods go even further and are defined as those where Māori themselves initiate the research (Bishop 2005). In this framework, indigenous peoples control their own research agenda.

When it comes to matters of research ethics, a Western approach is usually framed using principles such as autonomy and the rights of the individual, and the need to protect participants by ensuring confidentiality (Smith 1999). These assumed principles are problematic from an indigenous research perspective. For indigenous peoples, decisions are made within the collective, and these decisions may be subject to revision. Within VRE, this indigenous approach manifests as the need to engage in ongoing deliberation with those who are at the centre of the research, and negotiating decisions as collective. But when negotiating with the 'collective', decisions are not always straightforward. This is because agreements may be unstable (due to certain people being absent 'on the day') and decisions may have to be made 'in the moment' and 'for the moment'. You may find yourself taking risks or making decisions that you later, following reflection and with the benefit of hindsight, have to change. The following vignette provides an example.

I had been working with a multidisciplinary team of community-based clinicians for over a year. The team had become accustomed to my being around and for the most part, considered me as a member of the team. Every morning both sub-teams serving two geographical locations and comprising a core of three to six nurses, a social worker, a medical consultant and one to two mid-level trainee doctors would gather at a meeting called the 'huddle' – students of any discipline could also be present. Facilitated by any one of these team members with the aid of a whiteboard, they triaged patients' and/or families' need for home visits and decided the most appropriate team member(s) to attend. The meeting also served as a forum to discuss complex clinical issues and form management plans as well as to decide practical logistics of visits. With consent from team members, the researcher would film these huddles. It was the researcher's modus operandi to make the team aware the camera was running. On one particular and hectic Monday morning in the lead up to the huddle, multiple clinical interactions were taking place in sub-spaces within the room and across the room. There seemed to be more people in the room than usual. One of the senior nurses and a co-researcher in the team, realizing the complexities of what was unfolding, asked the researcher to switch the camera on. The nurse made it clear to me both verbally and non-verbally how keen she was to capture what was happening on film. I sensed her appreciation of the multiple interactions and complexity of what was happening in the room and felt the strong imperative for me to press the play button. However, as the huddle got underway proper, I noted there were two people present who I had not met previously. I was unsure if they had formally consented to the study and to be filmed or if they even knew it existed. Multiple thoughts about the pros and cons whirled through my head as I decided in a split second to switch the camera on and at the same time verbally voiced I had done so. Unsure if I had been fully heard, it seemed inappropriate to disrupt the flow of the meeting. Knowing I would be able to delete the footage yet the unfolding scenario could not be replayed, I pressed the play button. At the end of the meeting, I approached the two individuals to introduce myself. They turned out to be new medical registrars in the team. My initial attempt to explain my decision to film was fruitless. They appeared upset and angry and questioned whether I understood research ethics in an accusatory tone. They, of course, could not see my thought juggling as I, in the moment, had grappled with whether or not to film. From their perspective, I was a stranger in the back of the room with a camera who they had not met before. Moreover, as medical trainees they had, to date, 'grown up' with a positivist lens on research.

Noteworthy too here is that the requirement of Western ethics committees for researchers to guarantee participants' de-identification and confidentiality may be problematic and at times undesirable. The de-identification requirement may deny the research participant a voice and a face. For its part, the confidentiality requirement may mean that the researcher's voice is privileged over the voices of her participants, whereby sources of knowledge and information are either not fully recognized or misrepresented. Thus, Ermine and colleagues note that 'Western academic confidentiality rules and regulations stand in direct contravention of knowledge sharing as tenet of Indigenous worldview' (Ermine et al. 2004, p. 33). In contrast, and in line with indigenous ethics, VRE seeks to create common ground among clinicians, researchers, and patients. As Gubrium and colleagues put it, 'What happens to that [common] ground when participants are given pseudonyms or their names are deleted in materials produced through a research project that was meant to be empowering?' (Gubrium et al. 2013, p. e6).

Of course, institutional ethics applications will require a strong justification for not 'protecting' peoples' identities in particular contexts. Furthermore, taking a participatory approach does not relinquish us, as video-reflexive ethnographers, from our own accountabilities including paying heed to relations of power and how people are positioned in the research or project. This, of course, includes how you position yourself. Do you have a particular agenda behind the camera, when editing, or in reflexive sessions? How do you justify your agenda? And who gets to participate in the research and who does not? Whose voices (and faces) get heard (and seen) on camera and, critically, whose voices (and faces) are missing? Who gets invited to video-reflexive sessions and who gets to speak up in them?

Not surprisingly, Carroll posits that power is forever present, even in a democratizing research endeavour such as VRE. Indeed, she argues that power continuously shifts not only between clinicians and the researcher but is also mediated by the video camera and video footage as artifacts of power. It is this constantly shifting power, she contends, that is at the very heart of VRE. As a feminist researcher, Carroll argues for the need to be highly attentive and attuned to the relational aspects of her VRE research in the intensive care unit (ICU) by attending to experience, action and feeling, alongside knowledge (Carroll 2009).

> Writing about her ICU study, Carroll states,
>
> I experienced how easy it was during nonlinear editing using 'i-movie' and 'final cut pro' software to seamlessly join events that occurred across different times and spaces, and also to join different points of view that may have been disclosed in varying times and contexts. Collating different spaces and times for the reflexive DVD meant that the unique contexts which preceded and shaped interactions were prone to erasure or made largely invisible through their decontextualisation.... I was conscious of the large amount of 'agenda-setting' power I had as a researcher who not only filmed, but also then edited 'everyday' scenes from the ICU.
>
> *(Carroll 2009, p. 255)*

Carroll's is a feminist research approach, which advocates honesty between researcher and researched (Klein 1983, p. 95). Rather than taking a researcher-centric stance, a feminist approach advocates a collaborative approach with participants. Alongside collaboration, feminist video researchers have established the goal of social change as foundational to their methodology (Juhasz 2003, Carroll 2009). Feminist approaches position participants and researchers as both 'researchers and researched, observers and observed, and documentarians and the documented' at the same time (Kindon 2003, p. 146, Carroll 2009). Such a feminist approach gives rise to productive vulnerabilities (Collier and Wyer 2015). That is, when both participants' and researchers' roles ebb and flow, levels of uncertainty and vulnerability of both participants and researchers also shift and change. It is 'when both researchers and participants allow themselves to be open and vulnerable to confronting uncertainty huge potential for learning and increased agency is created' (Collier and Wyer 2015, p. 4)

CHRISTIAN THEOLOGICAL ETHICS

Besides indigenous ethics, Collier drew from Christian theology in her VRE study exploring the experiences of people with life-limiting illness (see Collier

2013). The biblical perspective of what it means to be human underpins her view of self and others. By viewing humankind, made in the image of God, as first and foremost a community of persons, human beings only know who we are by looking into the faces of others, but only 'by looking into the face of God do we know what it is to be human' (Watts 2004, p. 160). Or as Levinas puts it: 'In the human face, the Other expresses his [sic] eminence, the dimension of height and divinity from which he [sic] descends' (Levinas 1969, p. 262).

The implication of the foregoing is that every human being is to be treated with respect and compassion, and this principle is central to VRE. This principle translates into needing to be present for and to the 'other', where being present requires humility (Jasanoff 2003). Humility is 'the noble choice to forgo your status, deploy your resources or use your influence for the good of others' (Dickson 2011, p. 24). It is in this sense that Collier's humility manifests as 'ethics in practice'. For her, humility becomes the basis of how we pursue practical outcomes to situations as they unfold, prioritizing others' growth and well-being (Deleuze 1988, Spinoza 2001).

CONCLUSION: THE ETHICS OF RESEARCHER REFLEXIVITY

What all of the aforementioned approaches and frameworks have in common is the need for reflexivity. The three-layered framework described by Nicholls (2009) drawing on work by Chiu (2006) provides a helpful way of thinking about VRE reflexivity, and in particular, *researcher* reflexivity (Collier and Wyer 2015). While participants' reflexivity is the principal aim of VRE, researcher reflexivity is to be regarded as its 'mode of transport'.

Hence, and firstly, researchers are asked to consider the opportunities as well as the limits and opportunities that they themselves bring to the VRE collaboration. This involves researchers reflecting on their own positioning in all aspects of the research. This is *self*-reflexivity.

At the next level is interpersonal or relational reflexivity. This mode of reflexivity calls on researchers to evaluate their interpersonal encounters and capacities for developing relationships with participants. While VRE may be defined as a visual method, it should be clear that its absolute point of gravity is human relationships and relationship dynamics. Conducting such relationships well depends on our capacity for reflexivity.

Finally, there is collective reflexivity. Collective reflexivity asks researchers to consider how the process of the research as well as its design affects findings, how it structures outcomes for change and whether it enables learning. Ultimately, the issue comes down to this: is VRE able to inspire in participants (and in researchers themselves!) a growing receptiveness towards the world's complexity (Biesta 2015)? This question defines VRE, attesting it is not about producing formalized knowledge but about supporting people's growth and their learning in whichever way and direction serves them best.

The next sections of this appendix are devoted to specifying the research ethics guidelines that apply to VRE and providing an example of VRE data management.

VRE RESEARCH GOVERNANCE: ETHICAL AND LEGAL CONSIDERATIONS

This section outlines the legal and ethical framework within which we operate when engaging in video-reflexive work in healthcare settings. The document also addresses the specific issues that may emerge during the filming process and how we will ensure privacy and confidentiality for all clinicians and patients/carers that consent to be filmed.

Governance and ethical framework

Internationally: The *World Medical Association Declaration of Helsinki* (latest version 2013) pertains primarily to medical research involving patients; however, its principles apply also to research involving healthcare workers as participants: https://www.wma.net/policies-post/wma-declaration-of-helsinki-ethical-principles-for-medical-research-involving-human-subjects/

In Australia: Research involving human participants is governed by the *National Statement on Ethical Conduct in Human Research* (NHRMC 2007, updated 2015). In addition, research data is subject to the provisions of the Federal Privacy Act 1988 (www.legislation.gov.au/Series/C2004A03712). Within New South Wales, research is also subject to the provisions of the NSW Health Records and Information Privacy Act 2002 (www.legislation.nsw.gov.au/#/view/act/2002/71).

In the EU: As in Australia, in the EU research involving humans is subject to ethics approval from local nations' and universities' ethics committees. The recent introduction of the General Data Protection Regulation has implications predominantly for 'big data' research and data management, and its guidelines serve to support appropriate data sharing rather than limiting it. General data protection regulation (GDPR) affects the use of video data in research only in so far as such research might create a 'risk to the rights and freedoms of natural persons, of varying likelihood and severity, [which] may result from personal data processing which could lead to physical, material or non-material damage' (GDPR, Section 75). The GDPR recommends appropriate governance restrictions, and we provide examples of such governance principles below.

In sum, VRE research is to be conducted in accordance with your institution's and participating healthcare organizations' human research codes of conduct, protocols and policies. VRE research requires approval (and/or ratification) by the relevant institutions' human research ethics committee(s) before the study begins. Further, the research may also require approval from research governance units in the respective institutions and organizations involved.

Informed consent of research participants

Informed consent in VRE research is necessarily a process, due to the unpredictable (and potentially sensitive) nature of the video data being captured and the need to maintain the safety of participants. This entails both written and verbal consent being sought from participants at several stages throughout the research.

Understanding that VRE research may also involve other methods such as interviews, surveys and focus groups, the stages of consent required for VRE specifically pertain to participants:

- Allowing researchers to video their activity
- Allowing researchers to keep the footage
- Allowing researchers to show their identifiable footage to different audiences (which can include their colleagues, their care providers, their patients, other participants, other academic audiences and potentially the public)
- Agreeing to participate in recorded reflexive discussions, individually or in groups

Participants need to be informed as to the purpose, methods, demands, risks and potential benefits of the research, as well as their rights to refuse or withdraw participation at any point without reprisal. This can be communicated both in person and via specially tailored Participant Information and Consent Forms for participants to sign.

Wherever possible, all participants (healthcare workers and/or patients) should be invited to be informed and consent to participate prior to the study commencing or prior to any research activity taking place. Depending on the activity and location of the research, this is not always possible when videoing (for instance, if someone unexpectedly comes into frame in a busy ward to have a conversation with someone being videoed, or if someone comes into the video frame by performing some noticeable activity in the background). In such cases, the researcher should, if possible, pause the videoing to obtain informed consent 'on the spot'. If this is unfeasible, they should, at minimum, notify the person that they are being recorded, obtain temporary consent to continue videoing and then have the full conversation about informed consent immediately or as soon as possible afterwards.

The researcher must maintain an ongoing sensitivity to participants' feelings about the appropriateness of the videoing. Videoing is likely to be inappropriate in situations of crisis or distress for participants, and must always be stopped upon the request of those being videoed.

Where people are passing by, or 'in the background' and not extensively featured in the videoed footage, it may not be necessary to obtain their written consent to use the footage. However, wherever possible, their verbal consent should be sought, and their features should be blurred before showing the footage outside of confidential reflexive sessions.

With regard to the recruitment of patients, the involvement of their healthcare provider in recruitment requires careful consideration, as this may put patients in a position where they find it difficult to decline participation. On the other hand, researchers should, where appropriate, consult with clinicians before approaching patients, so as to avoid approaching patients who may be too unwell or vulnerable at the time.

Privacy and confidentiality of information and video footage: Legal disclosure

Any information obtained as part of a VRE project that can identify participants should in principle remain confidential by default. Participants may grant their participation on the condition that no information that will identify them is made public in any way. Researchers may also be required, for some hospital sites, to sign a hospital-based confidentiality agreement, preventing them from sharing footage with third parties.

If the researcher has health professional registration, he/she may be obliged to notify sub-standard practices either to management of the relevant health service or to the Australian Health Professional Registration Agency. This needs to be clarified up front to the health professionals' planning to be involved in the video research. They may be reassured however by the qualification that such 'extreme situation' has not occurred to any of those involved in video research to date that we know of.

For legal reasons, 'problematic footage' (capturing errors in practice) must be stored and retained by the researcher, even if it is not made part of the reflexive feedback process. Destroying such footage may put the researcher in breach of appropriate disclosure.

Barring legal subpoena, video footage will only be disclosed with participants' permission, and in ways and forums that meet with their approval. Special permission may be sought and may be granted by the participants, for the researchers to use video footage in forums outside of confidential reflexive feedback meetings (e.g. at conference presentations and academic lectures).

For any use of the footage, the request for permission should clarify whether or not participants wish their identities to be hidden (via blurring or pixelation), or if they permit their faces (and any other identifying information) to be shown. Formal 'media consent' forms may be used to obtain written (signed) consent from participants for the use of their de-identified footage in forums outside of the research.

Where information about non-consenting individuals is captured during the research (e.g. personal information about patients shared during clinical handover discussion), we will protect the confidentiality of this information. Any footage or recording that includes identifying information of non-consenting patients will be shared only with their participating healthcare providers and will be de-identified before being shared elsewhere.

Protecting confidentiality in data storage and sharing

Due to the size of digital video files, VRE researchers will need to set up secure storage (on institutional data storage systems, and/or password-protected computers and external hard drives) in order to store, back up, work with and archive their video data. Some researchers may wish to consider carrying their unsecure recording devices in locked bags for added security and/or to download footage from their recording devices as soon as possible.

Where possible, researchers will also need access to private workspaces in order to maintain the confidentiality of their visual data. They will also require locked storage space to secure their equipment, confidential paperwork and any data stored on external devices.

When sharing video footage as part of the research (e.g. during reflexive sessions or when showing footage to obtain consent to use it), researchers need to do so in private enclosed spaces, wherever possible, and to be conscious of the visibility and audibility, as well as the sensitivity of the footage shared.

What follows is an example of a VRE data management plan (our thanks for this section go to Dawn Goodwin, Suzanne Grant, Jessica Mesman and Marian Verkerk).

A VRE DATA MANAGEMENT PLAN

Assessment of existing and new data

The research objectives require qualitative data that are not available from other sources.

VRE is a specific methodology that requires participants to examine their own practices or activities. The process uses video recordings of healthcare practice to aid reflection and analysis that draws out all the contextual details that have informed activities. VRE provides a route through which participants can make improvements to their practices, but it first mandates a detailed analysis of those situated practices. Existing datasets are largely surveys of staff and patients (e.g. National Patient Surveys) that treat [the object of analysis] as a separate issue and do not contain the level of contextual detail necessary for analysis.

Information on new data

For these reasons, three types of qualitative data will be collected:

1. *Ethnographic field notes*: All field notes will be handwritten in a dated fieldwork notebook before being typed up in full and stored as Microsoft Word files. Files will be stored on the departmental filestore of the university. Once transcripts are completed, notebooks will be stored in a locked filing cabinet for the duration of the project (in case reference to initial field notes is required). When the datasets have been prepared for archiving, these notebooks will be destroyed as confidential waste. The appointed [research fellow] will be responsible for their safekeeping and disposal.
2. *Video data*: *Video ethnography* of key practices will be collected and will feature healthcare professionals, patients and families/carers. The digital video files will be stored in MP4 format for later analysis, editing and use during the video-reflexive sessions. The *VRE sessions* from each field site will also be video recorded and stored in MP4 files in the

universities' departmental filestores. These files will later be transcribed in full and stored as Microsoft Word files.

3. *Interview data*: *In-depth interviews* will be conducted with healthcare professionals, patients and carers. Interviews will be audio recorded and stored in WAV format, then transcribed verbatim as Microsoft Word files and stored on the departmental filestore of the university for the duration of the project (in case reference to the interview recording is required). Once datasets have been prepared for archiving, the audio files will be deleted.

The qualitative data software NVivo will be used to analyze, code and store all data and to facilitate analysis across different datasets. Themes and codes will be determined at project meetings and used consistently. The research fellow will code data and build up an NVivo repository stored on the university's departmental filestore. However, for project meetings and analysis, some data will need to be shared within the research team. This data will be saved in 'Box', which is a cloud-based storage facility provided by the university. It facilitates collaborative work once access to relevant folders has been granted. Box also allows granting access to researchers outside of the home university. Text-based data stored in Box will be encrypted Microsoft Word files, whereas video data will be encrypted MP4 files.

Metadata will also be stored in Box. This will include clear labelling of data type, field site, versions and dates. This will be collated throughout the project and stored as an Excel Spreadsheet on Box. It will be the responsibility of the research fellow to compile this record. Other research-related documents (e.g. methodology description, data management protocols, interview guides) will be stored alongside the metadata on Box. All members of the research team will have access to Box.

CONSENT, CONFIDENTIALITY AND ANONYMIZATION

Written consent of key participants will be obtained in advance of data collection. The consent process will clarify that data may be used in publications and participants will have the opportunity to decline this aspect if they prefer. However, as ethnographic studies are 'naturalistic' data collection, it is possible that people may enter 'the field', whilst data collection is under way (e.g. while patients, nurses and doctors who routinely work on a given ward may have consented, it is possible that a specialist doctor may be called upon to review a patient). In these situations, participants will be informed of the study as soon as possible and given the opportunity to consent or decline to participate. If they decline, all data in which they feature will be deleted.

To preserve confidentiality but retain contextual detail, all participants will be allocated unique identifiers. Unique identifiers will be formed using a combination of role, for example, patient/relative/nurse/doctor, participant number and field site (if relevant). Contextual information (indirect identifiers) will be recorded against these unique identifiers in case this becomes relevant to the analysis, for example, level of experience of a healthcare professional. In publications, and in preparing data for archiving, data will be thoroughly anonymized, removing all direct identifiers and study locations, and using generic descriptions in place of indirect identifiers. Unique identifiers and related contextual information will be stored, along with metadata, on Box and deleted after a period of 3 years from completion of the study. This period will allow for any further analysis, writing of journal articles and publication to be completed.

Ethnographic field notes: Observation and recording of field notes will focus only on those individuals who have provided written consent to participate in the study. Unique identifiers will be used when typing up field notes. Individuals are free to withdraw their consent at any stage until their data has been amalgamated into the analysis.

Video data: In line with other research studies employing VRE (Carroll et al. 2008; Collier et al. 2014), video data will only be gathered of individuals who have given prior written consent to being filmed, with individuals being free to withdraw their consent at any stage until their data has been amalgamated into the analysis. During data collection, video recording will be stopped if requested, and sensitive or inappropriate video data will be destroyed.

Interview data: All participants who consent to be interviewed will be given unique identifiers which will be used when interviews are transcribed. Individuals are free to withdraw their consent at any stage until their data has been amalgamated into the analysis.

QUALITY ASSURANCE OF DATA

The principal investigator (PI) will be responsible for overall quality assurance, with co-applicants being responsible for the specific activities conducted in their respective field sites.

We aim to appoint experienced ethnographers as research fellow; however, in the preparatory stage of the research, our approach to ethnographic fieldwork will be discussed and a detailed ethnographic data handling protocol will be developed by the research team so that a coherent approach (regarding field note-taking, level of detail, frequency of observation, approach to sampling and so forth) will be applied.

The research fellow will receive training in video ethnography and VRE. A detailed video data handling protocol will be developed by the research team during the preparatory phase of the project. Interviews will be conducted by the research fellow using a semi-structured interview schedule developed by the research team.

Responsibility for preparing datasets for analysis and archiving will rest with the research fellow, while their quality will be reviewed by the

PI and co-investigators (Co-Is). Interviews and VRE sessions will be transcribed by a professional transcriber, and their accuracy will be checked by the research fellow who conducted the interview or participated in the VRE session. The research fellow will have primary responsibility for coding the data arising from his/her field site, entering and coding this data within the NVivo repository. This process will be overseen by the PI and Co-Is.

Foreign data will be translated into English where it is necessary to facilitate collaborative analysis for use in publications and where it will be included in the dataset for archiving. Where translations are undertaken, a professional translator will be used and the quality and accuracy will be assured.

DATA STORAGE, BACKUP AND SECURITY OF DATA

Data will be stored in the file formats specified above in university, password protected and locations (as specified above). Data will be viewed at team meetings by the entire research team and will be encrypted and stored on Box. A filing system (which will include conventions for the naming of folders) will be developed to ensure the consistent organization and easy retrieval of data. Data files will be named according to the following convention: date/data type (e.g. field notes)/location (e.g. university)/researcher initials. Other research documents (e.g. reports or journal articles) will be named accordingly and identified by version number and creation date. These files will be stored on Box.

Using University-based storage means that data will be backed up automatically, anti-virus and firewall protection and software on researchers' computers will be updated regularly to ensure data integrity. University-provided cloud-based storage means there will be no need to email documents amongst the research team as all researchers, irrespective of location, will be able to access Box.

DATA SHARING AND ARCHIVING

For the ethnographic field notes and interviews, fully anonymized data will be deposited at the UK Data Service. However, due to the difficulties in fully anonymizing video data, the subsequent loss in quality of the data and the potential sensitivities involved in videoing health care, the video data will not form part of the archive for secondary analysis. Nevertheless, data underpinning research publications must be accessible according with publication guidelines. Therefore, where stills from the video recordings are used in publications, this limited subset of video data will be meticulously anonymized (e.g. by blurring faces and/or clipping the still to remove identifying features of the environment) and will be stored on University's research repository.

Strategies for safe data archiving:

- *Informed consent*: Data archiving, storage and reuse of the research data will be discussed with potential participants prior to consent being given. Specific consent will be sought to archive data: participants will be asked to sign separate consent forms for participation in the study (and the use of such data in dissemination) and for the archiving of data. Where consent for archiving data is not given, participants' wishes will be upheld.
- *Full data anonymization*: Data for which consent to archiving has been given will be further revised and edited to ensure that all identifying details (direct/indirect) have been removed. Careful consideration will be given at this stage to balance the potential loss of crucial contextual information (which would reduce the usefulness of data for future researchers) and the protection of participants' privacy and confidentiality. For longer-term data access, data will be converted to standard formats that most software are capable of interpreting, as per UK Data Archive guidelines (e.g. Rich Text Format for all textual data). Other metadata (e.g. interview guides, consent form templates) will also be revised and deposited to enable a fuller analysis.

Intellectual Property Rights

Ownership of intellectual property for the project will rest with the university, while ownership of copyright will rest with the PI, Co-Is and research fellow.

RESPONSIBILITIES

Responsibilities have been described in detail earlier. In sum, the PI will direct the data management process overall and oversee production and archiving of the dataset. The research fellow will produce the dataset and be responsible for archiving and metadata production. The Co-I will be responsible for the methodological training of all researchers.

REFERENCES

Australian Institute of Aboriginal and Torres Strait Islander Studies. (2012) *Guidelines for Ethical Research in Australian Indigenous Studies.* Canberra, ACT: Australian Institute of Aboriginal and Torres Strait Islander Studies.

Biesta G. (2015) Freeing teaching from learning: Opening up existential possibilities in educational relationships. *Studies in Philosophy and Education* 34(3): 229–243.

Bishop R. (2005) Freeing ourselves from neocolonial domination in research: A Kaupapa Maori approach to creating knowledge. In: Denzin NK and Lincoln YS (eds) *The Sage Handbook of Qualitative Research.* Thousand Oaks CA, Sage, 109–138.

Carroll, K., Iedema, R., and Kerridge, R. (2008). Reshaping ICU ward round practices using video reflexive ethnography. *Qualitative Health Research*, 18(3): 380–390.

Carroll K. (2009) Outsider, insider, alongsider: Examining reflexivity in hospital based video research. *International Journal of Multiple Research Approaches* 3: 246–263.

Chatterji AP. (2001) Postcolonial research as relevant practice. *Tamara: Journal of Critical Postmodern Organization Science* 1(3).

Chiu, L F. (2006). Critical reflection: More than nuts and bolts. *Action Research*, 4(2): 183–203.

Clark A. (2012) Visual ethics in a contemporary landscape. In: Pink S (ed) *Advances in Visual Methodology*. London: Sage, 17–36.

Clark A. (2013) Haunted by images? Ethical moments and anxieties in visual research. *Methodological Innovations Online* 8(2): 68–81.

Collier, A. (2013). Deleuzians of patient safety: A Video Reflexive Ethnography of End of Life Care. Sydney, University of Technology Sydney.

Collier A and Wyer M. (2015) Researching reflexively with patients and families: Two studies using video-reflexive ethnography to collaborate with patients and families in patient safety research. *Qualitative Health Research* 26(7), 979–993.

Collier A and Wyer M. (2016) Researching reflexively with patients and families: Two studies using video-reflexive ethnography to collaborate with patients and families in patient safety research. *Qualitative Health Research* 26(7): 979–993.

Deleuze G. (1988) *Spinoza: Practical Philosophy*. San Fransisco, CA, City Lights Books.

Dickson J. (2011) *Humilitas: A Lost Key to Life, Love and Leadership*. Grand Rapid, MI, Zondervan.

Ermine W, Sinclair R and Jeffery, B. (2004) *The Ethics of Research Involving Indigenous Peoples: Report of the Indigenous Peoples' Health Research Centre to the Interagency Advisory Panel on Research Ethics*. Saskatoon, SK: Indigenous Peoples' Health Research Centre, 1–272.

Gott, M., Seymour, J., Ingleton, C., Gardiner, C. and Bellamy, G. 2011. 'That's part of everybody's job': the perspectives of health care staff in England and New Zealand on the meaning and remit of palliative care. *Palliative Medicine*, 26(3):232–241. doi: 10.1177/0269216311408993.

Gubrium AC, Hill AL and Flicker S. (2013) A situated practice of ethics for participatory visual and digital methods in public health research. *American Journal of Public Health* 104(9):1606–1614. doi: 10.2105/AJPH.2013.301310.

Iedema R, Mesman J and Carroll K. (2013) *Visualising Health Care Improvement: Innovation from Within*. Oxford, UK: Radcliffe.

Jasanoff S. (2003) Technologies of humility: Citizen participation in governing science. *Minerva* 41(2003): 223–244.

Juhasz A. (2003) No woman is an object: Realizing the feminist collaborative video. *Camera Obscura* 518(3): 71–97.

Kindon S. (2003) Participatory video in geographic research. *Area* 35(2): 142–153.

Klein R. (1983) How to do what we want to do: Thoughts about feminist methodology. In: Bowles G and Klein R (eds.) *Theories of Women's Studies*. London: Routledge & Kegan Paul, 88–104.

Levinas E. (1969) *Totality and Infinity: An Essay on Exteriority*. Pitsburgh: Duquesne University Press.

National Health & Medical Research Council. (2007). National Statement on Ethical Conduct in Human Research. Retrieved from Canberra: http://www.nhmrc.gov.au/publications/synopses/e72syn.htm

Nicholls R. (2009) Research and indigenous participation: Critical reflexive methods. *International Journal of Social Research Methodology* 12(2): 117–126.

Smith LT. (1999). *Decolonizing Methodologies: Research and Indigenous Peoples*. London/New York: Zed Books; Dunedin, NZ: University of Otago Press.

Spinoza B. (2001) *Ethics*. Ware: Wordsworth Editions.

Watts RJ. (2004) What does it mean to be saved? *Evangelical Theological Review* 28(2): 156–165.

Wyer M. (2017). Integrating patients' experiences, understandings and enactments of infection prevention and control into clinicians' everyday care: A video-reflexive ethnographic exploratory intervention. PhD Thesis. University of Tasmania.

Index

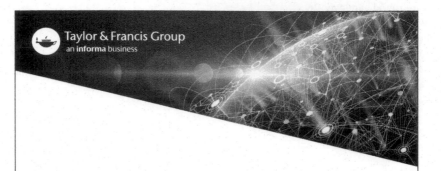